Topics in
Language
Disorders

Language in Context:
Listening, Reading,
and Writing

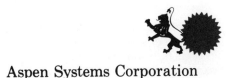
Aspen Systems Corporation

TLD Topics In Language Disorders

An Aspen Publication®

Publisher: Theodore Caris
Editor-in-Chief: John R. Marozsan
Editorial Director: R. Curtis Whitesel
Managing Editor: Margot S. Raphael
Associate Editor: Connie Braundmeier

Editorial Assistant: Ellen Gerecht
Production Manager: Paul R. Carlin
Advertising Manager: Joseph Del Master
Manager Fulfillment Operations:
Ernest V. Manzella, Jr.

TOPICS IN LANGUAGE DISORDERS is published quarterly by Aspen Systems Corporation, 1600 Research Boulevard, Rockville, Maryland 20850. Application to mail at second-class postage is pending at Rockville, Maryland and additional mailing offices. POSTMASTER: Send address changes to Aspen Systems Corporation, 16792 Oakmont Avenue, Gaithersburg, MD 20760.

Subscription Rates: $42.00 per year in the United States and Canada (four issues). Payable in advance. Subscribers may specify a particular issue to begin the subscription if desired. Subscribers in United Kingdom, Europe, Middle East, and Africa: Aspen Systems Corporation, 3 Henrietta Street, London WC2E 8LU, ENGLAND. Delivered subscription prices available upon request. Subscribers in Japan address subscription inquiries to Maruzen Company, Ltd., P.O. Box 5050, Tokyo International, 100-31, JAPAN.

Editorial correspondence (letters to the editor and manuscript submissions) should be addressed to: Editorial Director, TLD, Aspen Systems Corporation, 1600 Research Boulevard, Rockville, MD 20850.

Business correspondence (subscription inquiries, subscription orders, change of address, etc.) should be addressed to Fulfillment Operations, Aspen Systems Corporation, 16792 Oakmont Avenue, Gaithersburg, MD 20760.

Notices for change of address, including the subscriber's old and new addresses, should be sent to Fulfillment Operations, Aspen Systems Corporation, 16792 Oakmont Avenue, Gaithersburg, MD 20760 6 weeks in advance of effective date.

Single Copies: $13.00 each; enclose payment with order. Multiple Copies for Educational and Training Programs: Inquiries from bona fide educational programs concerning terms of sale will be answered promptly. Send inquiries to: Fulfillment Operations, Aspen Systems Corporation, 16792 Oakmont Avenue, Gaithersburg, MD 20760.

Advertising: Direct inquiries and correspondence to Advertising Manager, 1003 W. Front St., Red Bank, NJ 07701. Telephone: (201) 747-8658.

Copyright © 1981 by Aspen Systems Corporation, 1600 Research Boulevard, Rockville, Maryland 20850. All rights reserved.

Issue: Vol. 1, No. 2 ISBN: 0-89443-426-8
ISSN: 0271-8294
Printed in the United States of America.

Contents

Editorial Board

Doris J. Johnson, Ph.D.
Head, Program in Learning
   Disabilities
Professor of Learning Disabilities
Learning Disabilities Center
Northwestern University
Evanston, Illinois

James F. Kavanagh, Ph.D.
Associate Director
Center for Research for Mothers and
   Children
National Institute of Child Health
   and Human Development
National Institutes of Health
Bethesda, Maryland

Merlin J. Mecham, Ph.D.
Professor of Speech Pathology
Department of Communication
University of Utah
Salt Lake City, Utah

Rita C. Naremore, Ph.D.
Chairperson
Department of Speech and Hearing
   Sciences
Indiana University
Bloomington, Indiana

Bruce Porch, Ph.D.
Speech Pathologist
Veterans Administration
   Medical Center
Associate Professor of Neurology
   and Communicative Disorders
University of New Mexico
   Medical School
Albuquerque, New Mexico

Sylvia O. Richardson, M.A., M.D.
Distinguished Professor
   of Communicology and
   Special Education
Clinical Professor of Pediatrics
University of South Florida
Tampa, Florida

Jane A. Rieke, M.A.
Coordinator, Communication Programs
Experimental Education Unit
Child Development and Mental
   Retardation Center
University of Washington
Seattle, Washington

Joseph G. Sheehan, Ph.D.
Professor of Psychology
University of California
Los Angeles, California

Richard L. Schiefelbusch, Ph.D.
Director
Bureau of Child Research & Kansas
   Center for Mental Retardation and
   Human Development
University of Kansas
Lawrence, Kansas

Catherine E. Snow, Ph.D.
Visiting Associate Professor
Graduate School of Education
Harvard University
Cambridge, Massachusetts

Joel Stark, Ph.D.
Professor and Director
Speech and Hearing Center
Department of Communication Arts
   and Sciences
Queens College of the City University
   of New York
Flushing, New York

David A. Stumpf, M.D., Ph.D.
Director of Pediatric Neurology
Associate Professor of Pediatrics
   and Neurology
University of Colorado Health
   Sciences Center
Denver, Colorado

Geraldine P. Wallach, Ph.D.
Associate Professor
Department of Communication
   Disorders
Emerson College
Boston, Massachusetts

Joanna P. Williams, Ph.D.
Professor of Psychology and
   Education
Department of Psychology
Teachers College, Columbia
   University
New York, New York

Rhonda S. Work, M.A.
Consultant, Speech and
    Language Impaired
Bureau of Education for
    Exceptional Students
Florida Department of
    Education
Tallahassee, Florida

David E. Yoder, Ph.D.
Professor and Director of Clinics
Department of Communicative
    Disorders
University of Wisconsin—Madison
Madison, Wisconsin

Naomi Zigmond, Ph.D.
Professor
Director of Special Education Program
School of Education
Research Associate
Learning Research and Development
    Center
University of Pittsburgh
Pittsburgh, Pennsylvania

Letters to the Editor

All letters to the editor should be addressed to Editor, TLD, Aspen Systems Corporation, 1600 Research Boulevard, Rockville, MD 20850. Unless otherwise stated, we assume that letters addressed to the editor are intended for publication with your name and affiliation. As many letters as possible will be published. When space is limited and we cannot publish all letters received, we will select letters reflecting the range of opinions and ideas received. If a letter merits a response from an author or the editor, we will obtain a reply and publish both letters.

From the Editor

Reading maketh a full man,
Conference a ready man,
And writing an exact man.

> Francis Bacon (1561–1626)
> Dedication to the Essays
> Of Studies

The search for proficiency in reading, speaking, and writing skills obviously is not new, as Bacon's comments attest. In the second issue of *Topics in Language Disorders* (TLD) the search is continued for answers to both the theoretical and clinical issues facing professionals working with children and adults with language disorders. Again, we will look at language function within a transdisciplinary model.

Those who work daily with the "puzzle" children (e.g., the good speaker but poor reader; the good reader but poor speaker" or the good speaker and reader but poor writer) will find much information in this issue to assist in the identification and treatment of such children. Much of the research support for viewpoints taken by the authors in this issue and TLD 1:1 may lead to new ways of thinking about intervention strategies, especially the use of meta-comprehension instructional strategies.

This issue commences with an overview by Nelson, who suggests a comprehensive language intervention program for reading disabilities, language disorders, and written language dysfunction. She reports on successful strategies used in classroom settings while questioning some basic assumptions about intervention procedures. Nelson raises questions about a commonly held assumption that there is a clear ontogenetic sequence of development that may be observed in the acquisition of language from listening to speaking to reading to writing. She contrasts such an assumption with an alternate view that holds that developing skills may be used to facilitate skills that appear to be disordered. She notes

recent research that appears to support the notion that production can precede comprehension developmentally for some cognitively difficult tasks.

Nelson concludes that "normal language users seem to acquire . . . multilevel strategies and the ability to shift among them as the situation dictates, with little formal instruction. However, the child with a language learning disorder often does not." (p. 9). Finally, she suggests that we need not be constrained to intervene through the use of highly structured activities alone that focus on the form of the language or through the use of naturalistic activities alone that focus on content and use. Perhaps the activities can be fitted to the individual rather than the individual fitted to the activities. Nelson seems to suggest that there is no need for clinician and client to walk down the halls of time bonded together in a highly structured, and perhaps inappropriate, program. Nor does there seem to be a need for educator and child to be involved only in so-called naturalistic procedures.

Jenkins and Heliotis provide a current review of reading comprehension instruction and discuss the theoretical and practical issues that arise when there is an attempt to deal with the disparate findings from behavioral and cognitive psychology. They address the issue of "bottom-up" processing, or as they would term it, "analysis of comprehension skills," used by behavioral researchers. However, they also note recent studies that appear to support a "top-down" model of comprehension. The Jenkins and Heliotis article can be placed into juxtaposition with the Roth and Perfetti article ("A Framework for Reading, Language Comprehension, and Language Disability," TLD 1:1, December 1980, pp. 15–27) and the Pearson and Spiro article ("Toward a Theory of Reading Comprehension Instruction," TLD 1:1, December 1980, pp. 71–89). Each of these concern the possible interpretations by the reader of events portrayed in the text. Each article stresses, in differing ways, the importance of both context in the comprehension of the text and "world knowledge" or mental schemata that must interact with textual cues to create meaning.

For a view from the preschool bridge, the reader may wish to contrast the article by Sawyer and Lipa, entitled "The Route to Reading: A Perspective," and the article by Reid, "Child Reading: Readiness or Evolution?" Sawyer and Lipa define reading as the ability to respond to printed language and focus on reading as a communication process. They identify reading behavior as a product of the individual's various perceptual and cognitive ability levels, linguistic ability, expectations regarding interactions in society, and mastery of specific reading task demands. Theirs is an interactive view of reading. The inability of disabled readers to organize information and to process that information within a sociolinguistic context is stressed. Hemispheric specialization and the consequences of that specialization for reading are delineated. Case studies provide evidence not only of the inability to learn to read, but the inability to read to learn. Finally, Sawyer and Lipa question the value of reading research based on correlational studies. They point to the need to look at observable reading behaviors and the early identification of "at risk" children.

In contrast, Reid takes to task the concept of *readiness*, and espouses an "active" child model. For readers reared during the Ilg and Ames period, Reid comments on the possible harm such "readiness" testing, training, and postponement of the teaching of reading itself may have caused. She cites the need to use current research on learning and schema theory, whether it be spoken, read, or written langage, which must be related to past experiences. Reid reiterates that reading begins with the child's acquiring spoken language, commenting that in order for children to differentiate graphic symbols, those symbols must be mapped onto speech sounds. She emphasizes

that learning to speak, read, and write requires that the individual attend, select, organize, encode, rehearse, and retrieve information through a mix of current and past learning.

For many readers, attempting to deal substantively with disorders of written expression raises new questions because this may not have been perceived as an area of concern. Litowitz explores the nature of writing and provides significant information related to the alphabetic-phonetic writing system. She stresses the indirect, abstract way in which a writer interacts with his or her world. There are three groups of problems (a) deficits in underlying processes required for writing, (b) deficits in the complexities inherent in written representation, and (c) deficits related to instructional procedures. Litowitz cites the similarities and differences between the spoken language code and the written language code. Within a "bottom-up" model of processing, Litowitz reports that "writing requires analysis of those units in the acoustic stream which correspond to already established units in the visual graphemic system" (p. 7). Comparisons are drawn in terms of how different curricula in reading influence spelling by suggesting preferred strategies. Again, use of commonly accepted instructional programs, whether reading series, oral language intervention strategies, or individually designed remediation procedures, can effect the development of appropriate or inappropriate cognitive strategies by the language disordered individual. The reader may be interested in the focus on *authoring* (e.g., the ability to express ideas). Litowitz reports that both normal and disordered children have difficulty with "authorship" for many reasons, particularly because the receiver of the written word is an "absent other." Authors require audiences, but the act of writing must be done alone. Speakers also require listeners, but the act of speaking is one of interaction.

Writing requires deliberate analytic action, whereas speaking may deal with more global, less specific concepts or actions.

Silverman, Zigmond, Zimmerman, and Vallecorsa address the growing concern that language and learning disabled children be provided instruction not only in the necessary skills in reading, but also in writing. Noting that writing is perhaps "the most sophisticated form of language" and that the "generation of ideas" rather than the mechanics of writing should be the central theme, the authors provide salient suggestions for remediation. They report that while writing instruction is cited as a priority area in both special and regular education, it would appear to be a seldom practiced skill in the schools. Only 5% of instructional time is used for the writing of a child's own ideas. In essence, spoken language is advocated as a method of introducing creative writing tasks. Intervention strategies which center on the provision of cues and of organizing principles are stressed.

The generation of questions during an oral language period between instructor and student is recommended, with such questions answered in the written output phase. As children are assisted in developing organizational strategies, meta-comprehension and meta-cognitive strategies appear to develop. It might be valuable to examine the impact of practice under a carefully planned intervention program, using spoken language to enhance written language skills.

In this world of written, read, and spoken words, adults admire the lucid speaker, the skilled reader, and the carefully crafted written message. Language in context . . . how may professionals help those to whom these skills come less easily? This issue provides many questions and some answers. Professionals need both in our quest!

Katharine G. Butler, Ph.D.
Editor

An Eclectic Model of Language Intervention for Disorders of Listening, Speaking, Reading, and Writing

Nickola Wolf Nelson, Ph.D.
Speech and Language Consultant
  Specialist
Berrien County Intermediate School
  District
Berrien Springs, Michigan

THE CURRENT SWING back to basics in the field of general education is curiously out of phase with the trend toward insistence on naturalistic approaches to language intervention with language disordered children. This presents some unique challenges to professionals in the fields of special education and rehabilitation. Alternative views of what must be learned and of the processes involved in learning, storing, and using it have sometimes led to confusion. Dramatic shifts have occurred between emphasis on the etiology and symptoms of language disorders, between assessment and intervention strategies, between perceptual strategies and cognitive schemata affected, and between structured analytic and natural spontaneous approaches that might be applied in an intervention program.

0271-8294/81/0012-0001$2.00
© 1981 Aspen Systems Corporation

2

DEVELOPMENT OF AN ECLECTIC MODEL

The purpose of this article is to suggest that the best theoretical model for integrating apparently conflicting viewpoints regarding language intervention is eclectic. Without a model, program planning depends on buying the latest prepackaged curriculum. Alternative approaches that depend heavily on either a structured behavioristic model or an experiential naturalistic one are also limited. For example, structured behavioristic programs might teach isolated skills well but fail to relate them to comprehensive functioning. On the other hand, totally naturalistic approaches might merely replicate a setting in which the child has already had difficult learning language normally.

The eclectic model described in this article is based on a reanalysis of shifting assumptions about language disorders and intervention strategies. It has been developed to facilitate language acquisition among children who have shown restricted ability to learn language normally. This particular eclectic model has been applied in several classrooms for learning and language impaired (LLI) children in Berrien County, Michigan. It can also be used as a basis for inservice training of multidisciplinary professionals who bring differing backgrounds and emphasis to the intervention process.

REANALYZING OLD ASSUMPTIONS

Professionals who are charged with putting theory into practice operate with sets of basic assumptions. Such assump-

tions provide the undergirding for intervention models and affect their implementation. Periodically, to keep theory consonant with empirical evidence, it is necessary to reanalyze those assumptions. Four such reanalyses follow.

Assumptions on the nature of the population

a. Language disorders are closely related to specific etiologic conditions and vary accordingly; or the alternate assumption,
b. The population of language disordered children is etiologically homogeneous.

Part of the confusion regarding these assumptions is related to alternate uses of the terms *language disorder*, *language delay*, *language deviation*, and *language disability*. Sometimes the terms are used descriptively to highlight symptoms of a child's handicap, and sometimes they are used to signify a diagnostic entity (Bloom & Lahey, 1978). Problems arise when the differing applications of the terms are not made clear, particularly in reports of research on language disordered children. When children are selected for study of some aspect of language behavior based on a common diagnostic label but the dimensions of their current abilities are not described, it is difficult to determine the range of applicability of the research findings.

Historically descriptions of language disorders in children have been strongly linked to the medical model, in which particular etiologic conditions are felt to cause specific kinds of symptomatic disability. More recently the focus has shifted from diagnostic conditions to language systems. This is largely because of problems in establishing clear patterns of communicative behavior that can be reliably predicted for such diagnostic categories as autism (Cunningham & Dixon, 1961), cerebral palsy (Irwin & Hammill, 1965), Down's syndrome (Evans & Hampson, 1968), and learning disabilities (Atchison & Canter, 1979). At the same time that individual differences have tended to stand out *within* diagnostic categories, differences *between* such diagnostic categories as autism and childhood aphasia (Baker, Cantwell, Rutter, & Bartak, 1976), autism and mental retardation (DeMyer, 1976; Rutter, 1968), and mental retardation and normal development (Lackner, 1976) have tended to blur. Clearly, problems arise if etiologic categories are used exclusively as a basis for the development of intervention programs.

On the other hand, the development of a model for language intervention that can be expected to apply only to a single child is not efficient either. It ought to be possible to build a model that will provide a comprehensive, yet flexible framework, which can capitalize on general knowledge about language development and language disorders while providing direct opportunities for individualization.

Assumptions on using the components of language for assessment and intervention

a. Assessment tasks define language and can be directly translated into intervention tasks; or the alternate assumption,

b. Structured assessment tasks fail to tap the rich interaction of the components of language and provide little useful information.

The first assumption assumes that relative performance on specific tasks used in assessment should determine the kinds of tasks used in the intervention process. This approach is probably most evident in programs aimed at developing specific abilities using the subtest tasks of the *Illinois Test of Psycholinguistic Abilities* (ITPA) after it was published by Kirk, McCarthy, and Kirk (1964, revised 1968). In the specific abilities approach, the ITPA and other tests are used to identify a profile of relative abilities and disabilities for an individual child. Then a decision must be made whether to teach *to* a child's major area of disability or around it (Johnson & Myklebust, 1967). When a decision is made to teach *to* a disability area, intervention programs using this model may lead to recommendations for training children based on the ITPA subtests which yield the lowest scores. For example, children who score low on the Auditory Memory and Verbal Expression subtests may be asked to perform such tasks as repeating longer series of digits or making more "It's (a) N/Adj" statements about blocks and cups. When it is decided to teach *around* a disability area, a child whose visual subtests are much stronger than the auditory ones may be taught reading with a program which relies completely on developing a sight word vocabulary and avoids any reliance on phonics.

4

Psycholinguistic training

The efficacy of such "psycholinguistic training" of specific abilities has been seriously questioned by Hammill and Larsen (1974) in a review of 38 studies using the ITPA as a criterion for improvement. Lund, Foster, and McCall-Perez (1978) provided a reanalysis of the 38 studies and identified several weaknesses in the earlier review. However, many questions remain about the effectiveness of using a specific abilities model as a basis of language intervention (Bloom & Lahey, 1978; Bortner, 1971; Hammill & Larsen, 1978). On the other hand, psycholinguistic training and training based on the ITPA are not the same.

A better definition of a psycholinguistic-based training program might include recognition of the need to develop skills for using the various components of language—phonology, morphology, syntax, semantics, and pragmatics—within a cognitive framework. A task analysis of the 12 ITPA subtests shows them to be highly loaded on semantics, with only grammatic closure providing the briefest sample of morphological and syntactic abilities. Only the auditory closure and sound blending tasks tap limited aspects of phonological processing. Pragmatics is not a part of the ITPA test model. A truly "psycholinguistic" assessment and intervention program should cover all components of language and its use.

Assessment techniques

It is unlikely that any one test can effectively encompass all aspects of psycholinguistic behavior. Rather, a comprehensive language evaluation usually includes a broad sampling of communicative behaviors using one or more standardized assessment tools. This is followed by further testing in areas hypothesized to be particularly involved in the disorder.

However, formalized assessment has generally been questioned too, and it is in the second version of the second set of assumptions.

Muma (1978), in particular, has suggested a critical reanalysis of the use of standardized assessment techniques. Certainly it does not take many administrations of almost any test for the experienced professional to recognize its limitations. However, professionals in the schools, particularly, legally depend on validated measures of language to determine eligibility for special programs for handicapped children under PL 94-142. These should be supplemented, of course, by using such procedures for systematic observation of spontaneous language behavior as those described by Lee (1974), Tyack and Gottsleben (1976), Muma (1978), and McLean and Snyder-McLean (1978). However, there are also times during the establishment of assessment hypotheses that performance on an informal task such as repetition of digits can signal the need for observing syntax and phonological processing more closely. This does not mean that digit span provides a valid measure of short-term memory in its complexity or that recalling sequences of words should be a specific task to be used in the intervention process. However, recognition of the frequent *association* of such short-term memory problems with problems of syntax and morphology can indicate that further assessment is needed in those areas. It is important that the differences among screening procedures, assessment procedures, and intervention procedures not be confused.

Relating assessment and training

Although assessment tasks themselves usually should not be translated directly into intervention tasks, the entire comprehensive evaluation must lead not only to a determination of whether a child qualifies for special programming but also to an establishment of areas that need greater attention in the intervention process. Educators must control their professional tendencies to focus both assessment and intervention procedures on the current "hot" issues rather than on children's needs. For example, before the 1960s, the focus was on articulation. After Chomsky (1957, 1965) the focus shifted to syntax (Gray & Ryan, 1973; Miller & Yoder, 1972), then semantics (MacDonald, 1976; Miller & Yoder, 1976), and now pragmatics (McLean & Snyder-McLean, 1978; Miller, 1978), with cognition (Rice, 1980) on the horizon. Surely the needs of children have not changed so much. Rather, theories have affected how professionals observe children. If educators are not

If educators are not careful, children whose patterns of abilities and disabilities do not fit the latest vogue will not receive the individualized programs they need.

careful, children whose patterns of abilities and disabilities do not fit the latest vogue will not receive the individualized programs they need.

Assumptions on the relationships between perception and cognition

a. Auditory perceptual deficits precede and probably cause many higher order language deficits and should be the primary focus of a structured intervention program; or the alternate assumption,

b. Holistic cognitive processes exert a primacy role over perception, and isolating aspects of language processing from natural contexts in intervention is meaningless and useless.

If a language intervention model is to be developed for children whose primary impairments are in listening, speaking, reading, and writing, educators should carefully observe the language systems of such children (including those labeled as *learning disabled* and *language learning impaired*). The children identified for the Berrien County, Michigan classrooms for LLI children include those who exhibit phonological production, discrimination, and sequencing problems; whose mean length of utterance may be shortened, particularly during the preschool years; whose syntax shows omissions or transpositions of early developing forms, perhaps in combination with later developing forms; and whose prereading, reading, and reading-comprehension skills develop slowly. However, the general intellectual functioning and comprehension abilities of most of these children are relatively

6

intact. Within limits they seem to be able to handle the content of messages better than the form. For example, in speaking, although content may be maintained, form may be restricted. Semantically redundant structural markers, such as inflectional morphemes and auxiliary verbs, tend to drop out, especially when the pragmatic implications of the context are heavy.

Auditory processing deficits

One suggested explanation for many of these phonological, morphological, and syntactic symptoms is that they are caused by a more basic auditory processing deficit. In research summarized in collections edited by Keith (1977) and by Rupp and Stockdell (1980), a prevalence of problems in handling auditory sequential input, particularly at higher rates of speed, against a background of noise, or in the face of competing, dichotic, or alternating messages has been identified. In some cases a diagnosed neurological pathology can account for performance problems on such measures of central auditory processing, particularly when the disability has been acquired (Duane, 1977; Kimura, 1961). In others, neurodevelopment delay is assumed, and in yet others, a history of early intermittent conductive hearing loss has consistently surfaced (Katz, 1978; Naremore, 1979). Although the frequency of the association of auditory processing problems with language disorders has not been questioned, the frequently assumed causal relationship between auditory processing problems and language disorders has been questioned.

Reasons for processing problems

The sequential nature of acoustic stimuli themselves makes it tempting to propose a hierarchy of processes leading in a linear fashion from reception to perception to conception (Myklebust, 1954, 1964). However, a closer look at skills that have previously been assumed to be strictly perceptual has led to the conclusion by some (Bloom & Lahey, 1978; Rees, 1973) that there is as much evidence that higher order language processing problems cause the difficulties on measures of auditory processing as vice versa. Wiig and Semel (1976) include higher cognitive and semantic process in their outline of skills for auditory linguistic processing. This, in addition to the fact that there is little evidence that direct remediation of perceptual deficits improves general language functioning (Bortner, 1971), again suggests the need to look further for a strong base for intervention program planning.

Constructivist view of processing

One option would be to take an opposite view of information processing. Rather than adopting the "bottom-up" view that reception leads, in a relatively sequential fashion, from reception to brief storage to perception to comprehension to cognition (and back down in the case of expression), educators could adopt a "top-down" constructivist view. This view states that cognition is the constant overall controlling factor and that what is already known more directly affects how people filter information and what is perceived than vice versa.

The constructivist view is intended to explain cognitive processes in general. Speech, as explained by the Stevens (1960) and Chomsky-Halle (1968) analysis-by-synthesis models and the Marslen-Wilson (1975) parallel-process model, is viewed as an interesting special case (Cooper, 1972). The overall cognitive emphasis of the constructive viewpoint is stressed by Smith (1973, 1975) and is currently being embraced by many educators studying child language and its disorders. Neisser (1967, p. 10) explained the central aspects of a cognitive-based explanation of perception:

Seeing, hearing, and remembering are all acts of construction, which make more or less use of stimulus information depending on circumstances. The constructive processes are assumed to have two stages, of which the first is fast, crude, wholistic, and parallel while the second is deliberate, attentive, detailed, and sequential.

Assumptions on the development of language in its modalities

a. A clear ontogenetic sequence of development can be observed in the acquisition of language in its modalities from listening to speaking to reading to writing which should be maintained in teaching; or the alternate assumption,

b. Comprehension does not necessarily always precede production, and later developing skills may even be used to facilitate skills that have been missed or are disordered.

The first assumption was explained by Myklebust (1954). However, almost any first-grade teacher will predict that children who have excessive difficulty listening and speaking will also have difficulty learning to read and write. Most special educators emphasize that the normal developmental sequence must be maintained in intervention as well. For example, Berry (1980) noted that preceding listening and speaking, the ontogenetic order of development includes the even earlier stages of nonverbal and prosodic communication.

The emphasis of the second assumption is only slightly different from that of a developmentally sequenced approach. It is that the commonly accepted relationships of comprehension before production and listening and speaking before reading and writing warrant a closer look, especially for LLI children.

Comprehension and production

A contextual component must be woven in to understand the complexities of the relationships between comprehension and production. Comprehension tasks usually require the recognition of incoming information in a context which supplies some clues about the meaning of the message. In the absence of the relevant situational context, construction and production of a message based on what an individual already knows may occasionally be the easier task. As Vygotsky (1962) and Blank (1975) have indicated, production can also precede comprehension developmentally for some cognitively difficult functions. For example, children learn to produce such linguistic tools of logical thought as the conjunctions "because" and "therefore" before they learn to comprehend logical operations.

8

Written language forms may also be used more easily than spoken ones in some situations. Consider the assistance that the written representation of perceptually difficult phonological sequences can sometimes provide. For example, in a telephone conversation that is completely understood until an unfamiliar proper name is inserted, the conversation may be interrupted momentarily while the name is spelled. Once the name is perceived clearly, subsequent uses are easily processed. In another familiar example, learning to read often is the key to helping a child who has previously substituted the /f/ for /θ/ phoneme sort out confusion between the two sounds and begin to say them correctly.

Structured language

Although the previous examples are drawn from normal adult or developmental behaviors, the second assumption suggests that violations of normal developmental order are sometimes valid for children who have been unable to acquire abilities in the earlier stages without special help. Such is the basis of the McGinnis (1963) association method, in which speech and language are developed through a synthetic approach. McGinnis developed her method in the 1920s and 1930s for children whose central auditory dysfunction was so severe that they appeared to be deaf. The method has since been adapted by DuBard (1974) and by Monsees (1972), who has labeled it structured language.

The association method and structured language approaches use reading and writing as a base for developing oral language. Children are first taught to associate individual letters with individual phonemes and then to blend individual sounds and letters into syllables and words. Finally children are taught to incorporate the smaller units into basic sentence patterns and transformations. In response to criticism that the approach is unnatural, Monsees (1972) replied that it "is admittedly and deliberately 'not natural,' and does not attempt to recreate or emulate the sequences and processes of first-language acquisition" (pp. 10–11). However, Monsees believed that the method is justified because for some children, "the choice does not lie between fluent, natural language, on the one hand and slow, labored language on the other, . . . but between slow, stilted language and no language at all" (p. 11). Although it was primarily designed for children who have little or no expressive language ability, the structured approach has also been suggested as a method for children who have more severe reading than oral language problems.

Written and spoken language

The assumption having to do with the uses of language in its various modalities is also concerned with the similarities of the processes involved. The traditional view is that written language is just spoken language written down and that an individual reads by decoding (or recoding) the written symbols into their auditory counterparts. This view has led to periodic discussion over the lack of phonetic representativeness of English orthography and suggestions that the spelling system be overhauled or at least that a phonetic representation should be used for an initial teaching alphabet. However, as Chomsky and Halle (1968) have stated, the value of the conventional spelling system is that it corresponds more closely to the underlying abstract level than to the surface phonetic form of the sound system. Goodman (1973) has also suggested that although some readers, especially in the early stage of learning to read, engage in the process of recoding graphic input as oral input and then decoding, such a step is neither necessary for nor characteristic of proficient reading.

The level of processing at which written and spoken forms of language coincide is in their reliance on multiple rule systems for the generation and comprehension (which may partially consist of re-generation) of messages. Skillful readers and listeners have at their option three cueing systems—graphophonics, syntactic, and semantic (Goodman, 1973). They are able to apply all three systems simultaneously and to shift focus among them as the context (structural and semantic) dictates. Both listening and reading are thought to involve sampling, predicting, testing, and confirming. Only as much sampling is taken from the physical representation as is needed to confirm or disconfirm predictions about meaning based on context and prior knowledge. Both perceptual and conceptual operations are used in the application of this multilevel strategy, and a consistent sequence of one before the other is difficult to detect.

Normal language users seem to acquire such multilevel strategies and the ability to shift among them as the situation dictates, with little formal instruction. However, the child with a language learning disorder often does not. That is a primary reason for the development of an eclectic model of language intervention.

DEVELOPING AN ECLECTIC MODEL

eclectic e-'klek'tik, i- *adj* !Gk *eklektikos*, fr. *eklegein* to select, fr. *ex + begein* to gather. 1: selecting what appears to be best in various doctrines, methods or styles 2: composed of elements drawn from various sources (*Webster's New Collegiate Dictionary*, 1974, p. 262).

An eclectic model that incorporates elements drawn from various sources appears to be best suited to integrating the sometimes conflicting principles in the four sets of assumptions discussed previously. Using the dictionary definition of eclectic, what may be the "best" in various doctrines, methods, or styles varies not only with the needs of individual children, but also with the sophistication of available sources of doctrines, methods, and styles. Based on current knowledge, the eclectic model must at least incorporate strategies for integrating the differing assumptions discussed previously regarding (a) language disordered children as individuals who may fit certain diagnostic categories, (b) assessment tasks and their interaction with the components of language, (c) processing as both a perceptual and a conceptual activity, and (d) uses of language in its various modalities as a product of the application of multiple systems of knowledge and processing.

10 **Language disordered children**

Returning to the first set of assumptions, the practical aspects of dealing with the placement of children in special programs necessitate a specific definition about the population for which any intervention model is intended. The domain of the model should be neither too broad nor too restricted. One way to avoid some of the problems mentioned earlier in using diagnostic categories to define the population is to adopt an alternate categorical system. In one such system, Bloom and Lahey (1978) have described language as intersecting systems within the categories content, form, and use. Language competence, or knowledge, is viewed as an integration of the three systems, with the integration serving as a plan for organizing the behaviors involved in speaking and understanding messages (Figure 1).

Descriptions of the relative degree of difficulty individual LLI children experience in each of the language systems may be more meaningful than whether the children are mentally retarded, hearing impaired, aphasic, or emotionally impaired. Current legal practices in the schools usually necessitate some separation by category. However, within each categorical program it may be more useful to alternate emphasis on the content, form, and use of language as the needs of children dictate. All children need some attention to the integration of the three systems. Mentally retarded children may require relatively more empha-

---

It may be more useful to alternate emphasis on the content, form, and use of language as the needs of children dictate.

---

sis on language content, emotionally impaired children may need more emphasis on language use and the integration of the three systems, and LLI children may require greater intervention emphasis on the forms of language.

A categorical description using the headings of content, form, and use should not become too simplistic. Consider that the three elements might be viewed as beads on a string. Even when one area is relatively more depressed than the others, the downward weight of one bead exerts a similar effect on the other two. The eclectic model described in the remainder of this article is primarily designed for children who experience greater difficulty with the form of language than with its

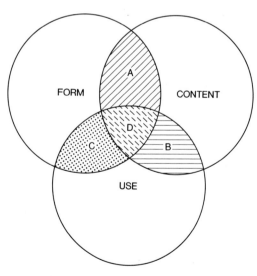

Fig. 1. The interaction of content, form, and use in language. (From Bloom, L., & Lahey, M. *Language development and language disorders.* New York: John Wiley & Sons, 1978.)

content or use. It therefore includes an emphasis on developing language form within an expanding framework of content and use. The broad limits of the population for which it is intended are described in the Appendix. The Appendix is a checklist of guidelines for diagnosis and placement in the special classrooms for LLI students in Berrien County, Michigan.

Assessment and the components of language

Returning to the second set of assumptions, a review of the checklist in the Appendix indicates that there has been no effort to specify *which* diagnostic tools must be used to identify children who would benefit from the program. What is needed is enough information first, to determine that a child has a severe enough problem to require intensive programming (i.e., the *quantitative* function of evaluation), and second, to determine the specific areas in need of remediation (i.e., the *qualitative* function of evaluation). A severe enough problem is defined in this case as discrepancy between potential overall ability and current skill in at least two of the component language systems, phonological, morphological, syntactic, semantic, and pragmatic.

To satisfy both requirements, especially the second one, one of the pieces of diagnostic information should be a spontaneous language sample. From the sample it should be possible to obtain at least a preliminary inventory of the child's probable linguistic competence or knowledge of the various rule systems for phonology,

morphology, syntax, semantics, and pragmatics and their use in spontaneous context. Qualitative information should also be obtained, using both formal and informal procedures, about the manner in which language is *processed*. For example, an adverse signal-noise ratio or competing messages may be used to identify performance factors affecting linguistic processing abilities.

Another piece of diagnostic information, and perhaps the most critical, is a determination of how the difficulties detected by direct assessment tasks are realized in the "real life" situations of home and school. Without this information, any intervention system will be severely limited. For example, although formal testing may show that a child has difficulty with such tasks as short-term auditory memory and discrimination, educators need to know whether there are problems of listening, speaking, reading, writing (and spelling), or thinking. Furthermore, if the model does not include a representation of *what* children need to know as well as *how* they are to learn it, the resulting intervention program will be without direction.

One way to conceptualize the content of what must be learned and the strategies for learning it is depicted in Figure 2. Figure 2 is an attempt to outline the relationship between the nature of knowledge and the nature of learning, pointing out both their distinctiveness and their interaction. The conceptual areas listed on the left of the figure are viewed as ultimate goals of maturity and the educational process. The skills listed on the right of the figure are viewed as the primary avenues of communication through which

12

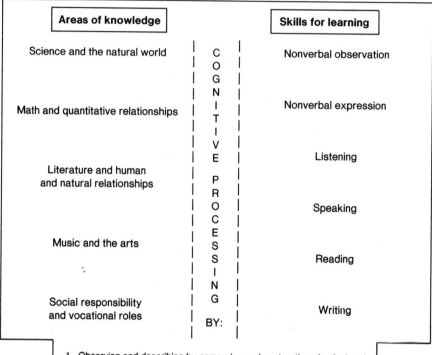

Fig. 2. A model for the differentiation and integration of knowledge and learning using cognitive processing strategies. (Adapted from Piaget, J. *The language and thought of the child*. New York: World Publishing Co., 1971; and Smith, F. *Comprehension and learning*. New York: Holt, Rinehart and Winston, 1975.)

developing individuals learn about the world. The cognitive processing, or problem-solving, strategy in the middle of the figure represents the manner in which knowledge and learning interact. The more one knows, the more one can learn,

just as the more one learns, the more one can know.

Language intervention programs usually do not even mention the kinds of conceptual areas listed on the left of Figure 2. However, language cannot exist without content and usefulness as well as form. Those two systems must be considered if a special program is to have any long-term effectiveness. Language impaired children, in particular, need to have a reason for developing the skills to communicate within and with the environment. Otherwise there will be little motivation for doing so.

Perceptual and conceptual processing

Returning to the third set of assumptions, perception and conceptualization can be viewed as having mutual effects, rather than one being prior (or primary) to the other. The arrows on a diagram of perceptual and conceptual processing should not have to go in just one direction. The "bottom-up" perceptual model does not provide an adequate explanation of how information is processed. However, the "top-down" model is also limited in its ability to explain the devastating effects related to sensorineural hearing loss and possibly related to even mild intermittent conductive hearing loss.

Educators must be careful not to commit the old error of applying what is known about adult cognitive processing too readily to the developing systems of children, especially those experiencing difficulty learning language for the first time.

Jones (1968) has said that children need more cues than adults to decode spoken or written language. Even normal children have processing difficulty in inverse proportion to the amount of acoustic or visual information in the stimulus. However, children whose auditory receptive systems are somewhat impaired are at an extra disadvantage for developing the cognitive structures that adults use for taking shortcuts in the perceptual process. Such children must be taught conscious strategies for processing auditory sequential information on multiple levels. Perhaps such children should be encouraged to engage in tasks thought to involve right hemisphere cerebral processing as well as the traditional activities of the left. For example, Edwards (1979, p. 196), in a fascinating approach to teaching drawing using a conscious cognitive shift, summarized the three main tasks of teachers as being (a) to "train both hemispheres—not only the verbal, symbolic, logical left hemisphere, but also the spatial, relational, holistic right hemisphere," (b) to "train students to use the cognitive style *suited to the task at hand*" [italics hers], and (c) to "train students to bring both styles—both hemispheres—to bear on a problem in an integrated manner."

Uses of language in its modalities

Finally, in returning to the last set of assumptions, regarding the sequence in which learning skills should be taught, there is no reason why some simultaneous attention to language production and comprehension in its various modalities cannot be built into the model of language intervention. Educators should use the intervention style suited to the task and then integrate resultant behaviors into the overall program.

Integration in intervention programs

Carefully designed teamwork between regular educators, learning disability specialists, and speech-language pathologists

14 can alternate daily between structured activities that focus on the form of language and more natural activities that focus on its content and use. In the Berrien County classrooms for LLI children, several different delivery systems have been implemented with varying time commitments by teachers of the speech and language impaired and teachers of the learning disabled. Although the training of those who deliver the services is important, the more crucial concern is that language disordered children have their needs met on a comprehensive basis.

Teachers of the learning disabled are generally more oriented toward classroom management and toward teaching the content subjects that appear on the left side of the outline in Figure 2. Teachers of the speech and language impaired are generally more oriented toward individual intervention and toward teaching the systems of phonology, morphology, syntax, semantics, and pragmatics that underlie the development of the communication skills on the right side of the outline. Without careful planning, when numerous time commitments become a problem, natural, content-oriented activities are often left to the classroom setting. Formal, structured-intervention activities are then isolated to the speech room. The danger is that such a lack of integration in the intervention program is likely to lead to a similar lack of integration in the child's knowledge and use of language.

Alternate focus on forms and functions of language

A conscious plan is needed for alternate focus on the many forms and functions of language. As symbolized in Figure 3, children are given several opportunities during the day to concentrate almost exclusively on aspects of the *form* of language while its content and use are externally controlled. Such structured activities are assigned to a specific time in the schedule and space in the classroom. Natural experience-based learning opportunities are provided in another part of the day and in less structured settings. This helps prevent the children from becoming confused about the differing behavioral and attentional expectations associated with specific tasks. It also provides a shift between individual or small group activities and whole group interaction.

Part of what identifies this approach as eclectic is that no requirement is made to develop a new form in its entirety before its use is encouraged in more natural situations. Function is seen as a facilitator of the development of form as well as vice versa. For example, notice of the effect on communication that fine adjustment in the form of language can provide may be encouraged in an experience-based science discovery activity. For example, shifting meaning with alternate uses of contrastive stress can function as a central mechanism toward early integration of new forms such as the copula "is"—"This water *is* salty; This water is *not*," and "This water tastes *salty;* This water tastes *sweet.*"

Modalities as facilitators

The various modalities are also viewed as potential facilitators of each other. Children with severe phonological disor-

DAILY OSCILLATIONS

OF LEARNING EXPERIENCES

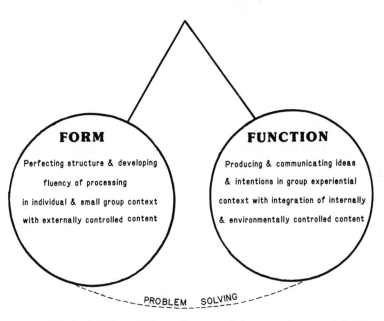

Fig. 3. An eclectic model for building daily oscillations of focus on form and function into learning experiences.

ders begin to sort out the sound system at the same time that they learn the multi-modality sound-symbol associations using McGinnis' (1963) techniques adapted by Monsees (1972). This helps them develop skills for auditory sequential processing for listening and speaking as well as the graphophonic cueing system described by Goodman (1973) for reading. Within the same day, development of the semantic cueing system is encouraged by having children choose their own sight-word vocabulary using words that are intrinsically important to them (Ashton-Warner, 1963).

Syntactic prediction is developed as children read storybooks that they have written (sometimes actually and sometimes in dictation). Each month a classroom newsbook is constructed from all of the cards which have served as the calendar for that month. Students also have personal newsbooks. News dictation intersects with verbal modeling of more mature syntactic structures as they are needed to convey fine shades of meaning. The books are illustrated by the children. Their transcribed utterances, along with teacher-modeled expansions, then become an ongoing language sample record book.

The pragmatic function of reading can also be encouraged by providing teacher-written materials through which children can learn about topics they have selected.

16

In this way children can read to learn at the same time they are learning to read.

For all of these activities, except for the structured language or association method techniques, spontaneity is to be valued more highly than correct form. However, during other parts of the day, target syntactic structures chosen for individual students can be developed using techniques such as those described by Gray and Ryan (1973) and Nelson (1979). The structure of those approaches, although currently rather unpopular, allows a high frequency of utterances formed with the same target structure to be elicited within a short period of time. The reliance on imitation and the relative freedom from need to concentrate on the content and use of language in the initial steps seems to provide the necessary element for acquiring syntactic rules missed developmentally. It also helps smooth out the fluency of language and provide a sense of "what sounds right," often missing in LLI children.

An important point is that children must be provided naturalistic opportunities within the same day to communicate freely without undue emphasis on using new forms. Spontaneous inclusions of new target structures are of course met with enthusiasm. An underlying principle is that all activities, both structured and unstructured, must not violate the multiple rule systems for communicative language. For example, if complete sentences are desired as responses, teachers and clinicians must learn to set up activities which elicit complete sentences naturally.

Teachers using an eclectic model are

Teachers using an eclectic model are encouraged not to feel guilty about using a variety of methods as long as there is ongoing evidence that the methods are working.

encouraged not to feel guilty about using a variety of methods as long as there is ongoing evidence that the methods are working. Evidence should show that individual objectives chosen for children, based on their comprehensive evaluations, are being met (Nelson, 1979). Pretesting and posttesting of all children in a classroom can also yield valuable information about the need for general program adjustments. Children themselves are provided feedback using wallcharts and individual notebooks as they acquire new sounds and structures. They are consciously led to develop multiple strategies for organizing and processing new information and for building strong associations for retention and recall of old information. Science and math programs are also chosen for their ability to facilitate cognitive organizational skills.

IMPLEMENTATION AND RESULTS

The first implementation of an eclectic model in a classroom for LLI children within Berrien County Intermediate School District (encompassing 16 local districts and approximately 615 square miles, and with a kindergarten to 12th grade public school enrollment of 41,307) was begun half-days at the preschool level in the spring of 1977. Pretest and posttest results are seen for the six children in that group in Figure 4. During the 1977–1978 school year, two half-day preschool sessions were provided. By the 1978–1979 school year, five other half-day preschool sessions were ˊadded around the county (including three taught by two teachers of the speech and language impaired and five taught by teachers with differing special education certification). In the 1978–1979 school year the first school-age classes were also implemented, with three in different locations for 6- to 9-year-old children and one for 9- to 12-year-olds. The data for one of those classes are presented in Figure 4. Since 1978–1979 the classrooms have remained consistently full (legal maximum of 10 students at any one time). One new level has been added in the largest district.

Children are moved from the LLI classrooms into regular education activities as soon as they are ready and for as many activities as they can handle. All of the classrooms are in regular elementary schools. Currently the five classrooms are taught by teachers with certification in the area of learning disabilities. In-class as well as individual sessions are provided by teachers of the speech and language impaired. Michigan has just passed a new rule which "allows" a teacher of the speech and language impaired to serve as the primary classroom teacher for school-age children who are severely language impaired. Therefore staffing options are now broader. All of the current LLI classrooms have, in addition to the instructional staff, at least part-time assistance from a teacher's aide.

The motivation for the Berrien County LLI classrooms stemmed directly from a recognized unfulfilled need for appropriate programs for specific children whose needs could not be met with speech and language intervention provided 2 to 3 times per week and resource room services designed for children with learning disabilities. The administrative support for the development of the programs has been an essential part of their establishment and maintenance. This includes such general considerations as funding with PL 94-142 flowthrough funds and such special considerations as hiring of substitutes for 1 or 2 school days per year. Thus the staff from the various districts can meet to share ideas.

In summary, when children are provided with a combination of structured and natural learning experiences which are separated and then integrated in the same day, they can make major strides toward acquiring the verbal and cognitive skills for learning. A problem in Berrien County has been that children's verbal I.Q. scores have sometimes jumped so much at 3-year reevaluations that staff have been unable to justify keeping them in the program. The staff may think that the children are not quite ready for a complete shift to resource room, regular classroom, and intermittent speech and language help—but that is a rather nice problem to have. In addition to positive changes in children, application of an eclectic model of language intervention has facilitated interdisciplinary cooperation. These LLI classrooms, and others like them around the country, represent the positive benefits of implementing PL 94-142 with enthusiasm, and other educators are encouraged to do the same.

18

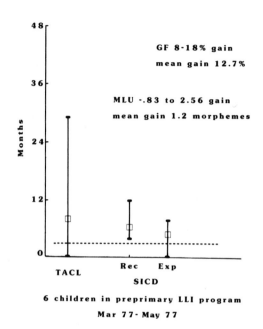

Fig. 4. Results of implementing an eclectic model with five classrooms of LLI children. Time between pretesting and posttesting is indicated with dotted lines. Solid lines indicate the range of months gained by students in each class from pretesting to posttesting. Open squares represent mean gains for the class on each measure. Gains in articulation ability and mean length of utterance (MLU) are also indicated. Test Key: GF = Goldman-Fristoe Test of Articulation (Goldman & Fristoe, 1969); TACL = Test of Auditory

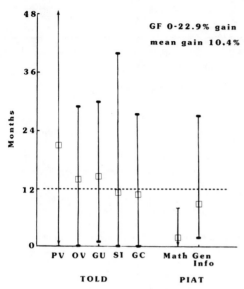

GF 0-22.9% gain
mean gain 10.4%

9 children in middle LLI schoolage program
Mar 79-Mar 80

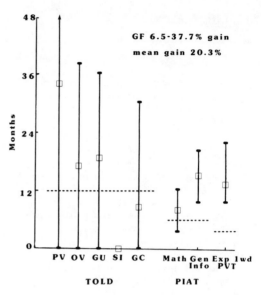

GF 6.5-37.7% gain
mean gain 20.3%

5 children in younger LLI schoolage program
Sept 79-Mar 80

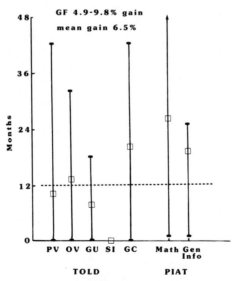

GF 4.9-9.8% gain
mean gain 6.5%

5 children in upper LLI schoolage program
Mar 79-Mar 80

Comprehension of Language (Carrow-Woolfolk, 1973); TOLD = Test of Language Development (Newcomer & Hammill, 1977); TOLD Subtests are picture vocabulary, oral vocabulary, grammatic understanding, sentence imitation, and grammatic completion; PIAT = Peabody Individual Achievement Test (Dunn & Markwardt, 1970); SICD = Sequenced Inventory of Communicative Development (Hedrick, Prather, & Tobin, 1975).

20   REFERENCES

Ashton-Warner, S. *Teacher*. New York: Bantam Books, 1963.

Atchison, M.J., & Canter, G.J. Variables influencing phonemic discrimination performance in normal and learning-disabled children. *Journal of Speech and Hearing Disorders*, 1979, *44*, 543–556.

Baker, L., Cantwell, D.P., Rutter, M., & Bartak, L. Language and autism. In E.R. Ritvo (Ed.), *Autism*. New York: Spectrum Publications, 1976.

Berry, M.F. *Teaching linguistically handicapped children*. Englewood Cliffs, N. J.: Prentice-Hall, 1980.

Blank, M. Mastering the intangible through language. In A. Aaronson & R. Rieber (Eds.), Developmental psycholinguistics and communication disorders. *Annals of the New York Academy of Sciences*, 1975, *263*, 44–58.

Bloom, L., & Lahey, M. *Language development and language disorders*. New York: John Wiley & Sons, 1978.

Boehm, A.E. *Boehm test of basic concepts*. New York: The Psychological Corporation, 1970.

Bortner, A. Phrenology, localization, and learning disabilities. *Journal of Special Education*, 1971, *5*, 23–29.

Carrow-Woolfolk, E. *Test for Auditory Comprehension of Language*. Bingham, Mass.: Teaching Resources, 1973.

Chomsky, N. *Syntactic structures*. The Hague: Mouton, 1957.

Chomsky, N. *Aspects of the theory of syntax*. Cambridge, Mass.: M.I.T. Press, 1965.

Chomsky, N., & Halle, M. *The sound pattern of English*. New York: Harper & Row, 1968.

Cooper, F.S. How is language conveyed by speech? In J.F. Kavanagh & I.G. Mattingly (Eds.), *Language by ear and by eye*. Cambridge, Mass.: M.I.T. Press, 1972.

Cunningham, M.A., & Dixon, C. A study of the language of an autistic child. *Journal of Childhood Psychology and Psychiatry*, 1961, *2*, 193–202.

DeMyer, M.K. Motor, perceptual-motor and intellectual abilities of autistic children. In L. Wing (Ed.), *Early Childhood Autism*. London: Pergamon Press, 1976.

Duane, D.D. A neurological perspective of central auditory dysfunction. In R.W. Keith (Ed.), *Central Auditory Dysfunction*. New York: Grune & Stratton, 1977.

DuBard, E. *Teaching aphasics and other language deficient children: Theory and application of the association method*. Hattiesburg, Miss.: University Press of Mississippi, 1974.

Dunn, L.M., & Markwardt, F.C. *Peabody Individual Achievement Test*. Circle Pines, Minn.: American Guidance Service, 1970.

Edwards, B. *Drawing on the right side of the brain*. Los Angeles: J.P. Tarcher, 1979.

Evans, D., & Hampson, M. The language of mongols. *British Journal of Disorders of Communication*, 1968, *3*, 171–181.

Gardner, M.F. *Expressive One Word Picture Vocabulary Test*. Novato, Calif.: Academic Therapy Publications, 1979.

Goldman, R., & Fristoe, M. *Goldman-Fristoe Test of Articulation*. Circle Pines, Minn.: American Guidance Service, 1969.

Goodman, K.S. Psycholinguistic universals in the reading process. In F. Smith (Ed.), *Psycholinguistics and reading*. New York: Holt, Rinehart and Winston, 1973.

Gray, B.B., & Ryan, B. *A language training program for the non-language child*. Champaign, Ill.: Research Press, 1973.

Hammill, D., & Larsen, S. The effectiveness of psycholinguistic training. *Exceptional Children*, 1974, *40*, 5–13.

Hammill, D., & Larsen, S. The effectiveness of psycholinguistic training: A reaffirmation of position. *Exceptional Children*, 1978, *44*, 402–414.

Hedrick, D.L., Prather, E.M., & Tobin, A.R. *Sequenced Inventory of Communication Development*. Seattle: University of Washington Press, 1975.

Irwin, O.C., & Hammill, D. Effect of type, extent and degree of cerebral palsy on three measures of language. *Cerebral Palsy Journal*, 1965, *26*, 7–9.

Johnson, D., & Myklebust, H. *Learning disabilities: Educational principles and practices*. New York: Grune & Stratton, 1967.

Jones, M.H. Some thoughts on perceptual units in language processing. In K.S. Goodman (Ed.), *The psycholinguistic nature of the reading process*. Detroit: Wayne State University Press, 1968.

Katz, J. The effects of conductive hearing loss on auditory function. *ASHA*, 1978, *28*, 879–886.

Keith, R.W. (Ed.) *Central auditory dysfunction*. New York: Grune & Stratton, 1977.

Kimura, D. Some effects of temporal-lobe damage on auditory perception. *Canadian Journal of Psychology*, 1961, *15*, 156–165.

Kirk, S., McCarthy, J., and Kirk, W. *The Illinois Test of Psycholinguistic Abilities*, (Revised Ed.). Urbana, Ill.: University of Illinois Press, 1968.

Lackner, J.R. A developmental study of language behavior in retarded children. *Neuropsychologia*, 1968, *6*, 301–320. Reprinted in D. Morehead & A. E. Morehead (Eds.), *Normal and deficient child language*. Baltimore: University Park Press, pp. 181–208, 1976.

Lee, L. *Developmental sentence analysis*. Evanston, Ill.: Northwestern University Press, 1974.

Lee, L.L., Koenigsknecht, R., & Mulhern, S. *Interactive language development teaching*. Evanston, Ill.: Northwestern University Press, 1975.

Lund, K.A., Foster, G.E., & McCall-Perez, F.C. The effectiveness of psycholinguistic training, a reevaluation. *Exceptional Children*, 1978, *44*, 310–330.

MacDonald, J.D. Environmental language intervention: Programs for establishing initial communication in handicapped children. In F. Withrow & C. Nygren (Eds.), *Language and the handicapped learner: Curricula, programs and media*. Columbus, Ohio: Charles E. Merrill, 1976.

Marslen-Wilson, W.D. Sentence perception as an interactive parallel process. *Science*, 1975, *189*, 226–228.

McGinnis, M. *Aphasic children*. Washington, D.C.: Alexander Graham Bell Association, 1963.

McLean, J.E., & Snyder-McLean, L.K. *A transactional approach to early language training*. Columbus, Ohio: Charles E. Merrill, 1978.

Miller, J., & Yoder, D. A syntax teaching program. In J. McLean, D. Yoder, & R. Schiefelbusch (Eds.), *Language intervention with the retarded*. Baltimore: University Park Press, 1972.

Miller, J., & Yoder, D. An ontogenetic language teaching strategy for retarded children. In. R.L. Schiefelbusch & L.L. Lloyd (Eds.), *Language perspectives: Acquisition, retardation and intervention*. Baltimore: University Park Press, 1976.

Miller, L. Pragmatics and early childhood language disorders: Communicative interactions in a half-hour sample. *Journal of Speech and Hearing Disorders*, 1978, *43*, 419–436.

Monsees, E.K. *Structured language for children with special language learning problems*. Washington, D.C.: Children's Hospital National Medical Center, 1972.

Muma, J.R. *Language handbook: Concepts, assessment, intervention*. Englewood Cliffs, N.J.: Prentice-Hall, 1978.

Myklebust, H.R. *Auditory disorders in children*. New York: Grune & Stratton, 1954.

Myklebust, H.R. *The psychology of deafness: Sensory deprivation, learning and adjustment*. New York: Grune & Stratton, 1964.

Naremore, R.C. Influences of hearing impairment on early language development. *Annals of Otology, Rhinology and Laryngology*, 1979, *88* (5, pt. 2), 54–63.

Neisser, U. *Cognitive psychology*. New York: Appleton-Century-Crofts, 1967.

Nelson, N.W. *Planning individualized speech and language intervention programs*. Tucson, Ariz.: Communication Skill Builders, 1979.

Newcomer, P.L., & Hammill, D. *Test of language development*. Austin, Tex.: Empiric Press, 1977.

Piaget, J. *The language and thought of the child*. New York: World Publishing Co., 1971.

Rees, N. Auditory processing factors in language disorders: The view from Procrustes' bed. *Journal of Speech and Hearing Disorders*, 1973, *38*, 304–315.

Rice, M. *Cognition to language*. Baltimore: University Park Press, 1980.

Rupp, R.R., & Stockdell, K.G. (Eds). *Speech protocols in audiology*. New York: Grune & Stratton, 1980.

Rutter, M. Concepts of autism. *Journal of Child Psychology and Psychiatry*, 1968, *9*, 1–25.

Slobin, D.I. *Psycholinguistics*. Glenview, Ill.: Scott, Foresman and Co., 1971.

Smith, F. (Ed.) *Psycholinguistics and reading*. New York: Holt, Rinehart and Winston, 1973.

Smith, F. *Comprehension and learning*. New York: Holt, Rinehart and Winston, 1975.

Stevens, K.N. Toward a model for speech recognition. *Journal of the Acoustical Society of America*, 1960, *32*, 47–55.

Tyack, D., & Gottsleben, R. *Language sampling, analysis and training: A handbook for teachers and clinicians*. Palo Alto, Calif.: Consulting Psychological Press, 1974.

Vygotsky, L.S. *Thought and language*. Cambridge, Mass.: M.I.T. Press, 1962.

Webster's New Collegiate Dictionary. Springfield, Mass.: G. & C. Merriam Co., 1974.

Wiig, E.H., & Semel, E.M. *Language disabilities in children and adolescents*. Columbus, Ohio: Charles E. Merrill, 1976.

22

Appendix

Referral and Placement Procedures for Berrien County Programs for Learning and Language Impaired (LLI) Students

When a child is being considered for placement in a classroom program for learning and language impaired students, the Special Education Director/Coordinator of the student's resident district assists in assuring that the following procedures have been completed:

1. The multidisciplinary comprehensive evaluation should include:

Psychological assessment demonstrating

- Potential functioning within or above normal intellectual ability as measured by instruments that do not rely exclusively on oral direction or oral expression (e.g., Leiter International Performance Scales, French Pictorial, subtests of WISC-R, less formal developmental scales), showing some of the following characteristics:
- Psychometric scatter (in most cases Verbal Scale scores will fall considerably below Performance Scale scores on the WISC-R, for example, although some verbally apraxic children may show higher verbal scale than performance scale scores);
- Major discrepancy (1 year or more) between some areas of psychological evaluation and some areas of language disability;
- Possibly depressed composite intellectual quotient (EMI range) in occa-

sional cases, but with some subtest scores suggesting normal intellectual potential;

- Eligibility for programming as learning impaired or severely language impaired as specified in state and local guidelines, possibly including attentional, memory, and information processing characteristics associated with childhood aphasia as evidenced by direct observation or performance on such tests as the Bender.

Language, speech, and hearing assessment demonstrating

- Oral/aural language which is clearly inappropriate (1 year or more discrepancy and/or greater than 2 S.D. below mean) for the child's level of intellectual functioning in two of the areas listed below. Both informal and formal (at least two of such tests as SICD, Zimmerman, Bankson, TACL, TOLD, PPVT, ITPA, PICAC, BTBC, SPLT, OLSIST, or others) test results should be used in making the determination:
- Phonological (every child should have recent results from a thorough articulation evaluation);
- Morphological and syntactic (every child should have a written spontaneous language sample and tape, with

100 utterances if possible. It need not be analyzed);

- Semantic (possibly including a PPVT and BTBC, but supplemented by description of the child's ability to combine words meaningfully and to have alternatives available for indicating shades of meaning);
- Pragmatic (usually not formally evaluated but determined by child's ability to use language in natural contexts to achieve various communicative functions such as providing just the right amount of information in conversation, staying on topic, knowing how and when to use pronouns, being able to comprehend and formulate indirect "polite" requests, and being able to switch communicative styles as appropriate;
- Hearing within normal limits as shown by recent audiological screening with an audiometer; however, some children with a history of recurrent middle ear infection are appropriate candidates for the LLI program. (Whenever more in-depth audiological testing is necessary, prior to IEPC the referring TSLI should assist the family in scheduling an appointment with an audiologist.)
- Teacher consultant assessment supporting a diagnosis of learning impairment (for school-age children);
- Occupational and/or physical assessment, if recommended during the course of other evaluation procedures (especially sensory integration).

2. Prior to IEPC, contact should be made with consulting, supervisory, and teaching personnel of the recommended LLI program. In some instances an observational visit can be arranged for the BCISD Speech-Language Consultant or others to determine if the LLI classroom program is an appropriate educational alternative to be considered at an IEPC: LLI classroom programs are located in Benton Harbor, Berrien Springs, New Buffalo, or Niles for preprimary children (3- to 5-year-olds); Benton Harbor, Berrien Springs, or Niles for school-age children (6- to 9-year-olds); and Niles for older school-age children (9- to 12-year-olds).

3. An IEPC to consider an LLI classroom program should include personnel in the following categories from both sending and receiving districts (if they are not the same), but especially those who have completed the diagnosis:

- Child's parents
- Psychologist
- Teacher of Speech and Language Impaired
- Sending Teacher and LLI Teacher

Others who are invited as appropriate are:

- Special Education Director/Coordinator
- Principal
- Teacher Consultant (especially if the child is school age and a TC diagnosis has been completed)
- Speech-Language Consultant for BCISD
- OT/PT
- Social Worker

Reading Comprehension Instruction: Findings from Behavioral and Cognitive Psychology

Joseph R. Jenkins, Ph.D.
Director

James G. Heliotis, M.Ed.
Coordinator, Learning
  Disabilities Program
Experimental Education Unit
University of Washington
Seattle, Washington

IN ADDRESSING the topic of reading comprehension, we have elected to examine research from the areas of behavioral and cognitive psychology. Given the enormous volume of work on the topic of comprehension, our review is necessarily selective rather than exhaustive. Also, we do not see work originating from differing theoretical frameworks as necessarily contradictory. In fact, thoughtful integration of selected components derived from behavioral and cognitive analyses should ultimately result in improved reading instruction. We anticipate that in the future reading programs will be developed which combine selected characteristics of applied behavior analysis (e.g., frequent and careful monitoring of student progress) with characteristics of direct instruction, along with insights into the identification of teaching content that emanate from cognitive psychology.

While research on reading has a long history (Huey, 1908), most early studies

0271-8294/81/0012-0025$2.00
© 1981 Aspen Systems Corporation

26

were descriptive and correlational. Later there were more experimental studies as psychologists turned their attention to this field. Even then researchers concentrated on issues related to perception and decoding. For example, the major reading controversy of the 1960s dealt with the relative merits of whole word versus phonics instruction (Chall, 1967). The lack of research activity in the area of comprehension could not be attributed to educational researchers' failure to recognize the importance of comprehension—no one needed to be convinced that reading is language comprehension. Rather, the explanation for the historical dominance of decoding over comprehension research can be traced to two assumptions held by many researchers and reading educators. First, basic skills in decoding were generally assumed to be prerequisite to understanding text. Thus, decoding was a major problem. Second, early analyses of reading assumed, perhaps implicitly, that once children could decode accurately and fluently, comprehension would automatically follow.

Many current reading researchers are far less sanguine about this second assumption and as a result are focusing more of their attention on issues related to reading comprehension. However, as with the early decoding research, much of the preliminary work in comprehension is descriptive and correlational. While experimental studies are increasing, relatively few researchers have examined variables which could be practically manipulated in instructional settings. Perhaps behavioral researchers, because of their philosophical orientation toward intervention, have taken more activist

roles in attempting both to identify instructional and motivational variables and to package empirically derived curricula for classroom use.

BEHAVIORAL RESEARCH IN READING COMPREHENSION

Behavioral research in reading comprehension has followed two major themes. The first stems from the application of behavior analysis procedures to ongoing classroom instruction while the second focuses on curriculum development. Several distinctive features relating either to student performance or to specific interventions, characterize the applied behavior analysis approach. One feature related to student performance is the regular and frequent monitoring of individual student responses using daily measurements and graphs showing results. Such monitoring provides teachers with information on each individual's (not just the group's) performance, thereby enabling teachers to make appropriate adjustments in their instructional program based on this information.

Moreover, the performance measures tend to be defined uniformly across days. The teacher is likely to record separately on a daily basis such indices as answers to factual, sequential, vocabulary, and inferential questions. This uniformity contrasts with the more common classroom practice of emphasizing different skills on different days, for example, teaching a main idea lesson on Monday, a vocabulary lesson on Tuesday, a pronoun lesson on Wednesday, a sequence exercise on Thursday, and so on. In one analysis of commercial reading programs, Engelmann and Steely (1980) reported that an average of 62 days passed between recurrences of a given topic.

Applied behavior analysts have favored consequence manipulations, such as varying reinforcement for correct responses, and secondarily used antecedent manipulations, such as modeling and prompting. In this way the conceptualization of intervention strategies for reading comprehension may be viewed as an extension of the principles of general behavior analysis. A final but significant characteristic of this approach is its reliance on previously developed, commonly used instructional materials and reading selections. Teachers generally superimpose a carefully designed behavioral system onto a situation where children are reading selections drawn from their regular program or from a supplementary series such as the SRA Reading Labs.

Comprehension researchers using an applied behavioral analysis approach tend to use uniform response measures daily; monitor and graph individual performance, or monitor and chart select interventions from a general behavior analytic model; and superimpose these interventions on widely disseminated, commercially available reading materials.

The second type of behavioral approach, labeled direct instruction, after Becker and Engelmann (1977), differs from the applied behavior analysis model in several important respects. One major difference is the emphasis on direct instruction in both curriculum design and teachers' presentation techniques. The direct instruction approach focuses not only on the content of the material presented—the selection of skills and teaching examples—but also on the initial introduction and sequencing of those skills and examples, the frequency with which practice items are introduced and reviewed, and the development of specific instructional strategies. Certain teacher presentation variables are also characteristic of a direct instruction approach, such as simple, clear, and usually scripted teacher directions; error corrections; and use of both group and individual responses.

Applied behavior analysis

Contingent reinforcement

Many researchers have examined the effects of contingent reinforcement on reading comprehension. The results of these investigations have not been entirely consistent, for example, the research of Staats and his colleagues (Staats & Butterfield, 1965; Staats, Minke, Goodwin, & Landeen, 1967). These investigators arranged for students to earn token reinforcers for correct answers on their daily reading quizzes. Token reinforcement produced improved comprehension in one study (Staats & Butterfield, 1965), but not in the other (Staats et al., 1967). Likewise, Camp and Van Doorninck (1971) found that comprehension was unchanged following contingent reinforcement procedures. However, more recent studies have reported positive effects for contingency management procedures (Hansen & Lovitt, 1976; Jenkins, Barksdale, & Clinton, 1978; Lahey, McNees, & Brown, 1973; Lovitt & Hansen, 1976; Roberts & Smith, 1980).

Consideration of the behaviors that contingent reinforcement is likely to

28

affect may explain why this intervention appears to increase comprehension in some situations but not in others. Introducing a reinforcement contingency will probably not provide students with new skills or strategies for comprehending text. Rather, access to reinforcers may induce students to use those skills they already possess. Analysis of reinforcement studies in which positive effects were noted suggests a motivational explanation. An example is the study of Jenkins et al. (1978), in which reading comprehension performance was examined simultaneously in a remedial setting and in a regular classroom. When learning disabled students were reinforced for improved comprehension performance in the remedial setting, their reading comprehension improved in that location. However, this improvement did not generalize to the classroom, even though the reading task there was similar. Only when contingent reinforcement was introduced in the classroom did comprehension performance improve in that location. Students in this study were probably already able to comprehend satisfactorily (even though this fact was not obvious from either their classroom performance or their test scores), but they did not exhibit this competency under normal classroom circumstances.

Lovitt and Hansen (1976), in contrast, went beyond strict reinforcement application. Students were carefully given reading materials and instruction that included daily practice on several types of comprehension questions and corrective feedback in addition to reinforcement for correct answers. A similar "intervention package," which included training in

word meanings, "focusing" on comprehension, and contingent points for correct answers to comprehension questions, resulted in substantial increases in performance on comprehension questions in the Roberts and Smith study (1980). Therefore, the substantial improvements noted in these studies (Hansen & Lovitt, 1976; Lovitt & Hansen, 1976; Roberts & Smith, 1980) could be a function of combined instructional and motivational factors.

Teaching comprehension-related skills

Other attempts to improve comprehension using applied behavior analysis have sought to influence comprehension indirectly by teaching comprehension-related skills. For example, the effect of vocabulary instruction on several types of reading comprehension tasks was evaluated in three experiments (Jenkins, Pany, & Schreck, 1978; Pany, 1978; Pany & Jenkins, 1978). Compared to indirect instruction (i.e., learning word meanings from context), direct and explicit vocabulary instruction consisting of synonym drill produced superior performance on all kinds of vocabulary measures. The superiority of the direct vocabulary instruction was also observed on sentence comprehension measures, but, importantly, *not* on overall passage comprehension.

The effect on reading comprehension of increased reading fluency has been evaluated with somewhat contradictory results (Dahl, 1974; Fleisher, Jenkins, & Pany, 1979). In the Fleisher et al. study, students identified as poor readers received training in rapid decoding. Though the reading rate of those students was increased substantially, their performance on reading comprehension measures was essentially the same as that of another group of poor readers who had not received rapid decoding training. In contrast, Dahl found a significant advantage in comprehension for students who participated in a year-long program that focused on increasing oral reading rates. The divergent results reported by Fleisher et al. and Dahl may be because of the longer duration and kind of fluency training used in the Dahl study. Dahl provided fluency training through a reading-in-context format while Fleisher et al. attempted to increase fluency through an isolated word procedure.

Direct instruction

A second behavioral front in the field of comprehension research is direct instruction. The most distinguishing feature of this approach is an attempt to teach "how to." An examination of workbook exercises and teacher-directed lessons from basal reading series reveals that "comprehension instruction" typically consists of opportunities to comprehend particular stimulus materials. The learner is rarely taught *how to comprehend*. For example, a teacher assigns a workbook exercise involving a series of passive sentences such as "John was teased by Mary," accompanied by questions such as "Who did the teasing?" Subsequently the students receive feedback on the accuracy of their performance when the workbook is corrected. Thus instruction might be characterized more accurately as comprehension practice with delayed feedback. While practice and feedback may be

considered instruction in some senses, they certainly do not qualify as instruction of the "how to" variety.

Durkin (1978–1979) documented that real *instruction* in comprehension is something of an endangered species. She conducted a large-scale observational study of classroom reading instruction. *Comprehension instruction* was defined as doing or saying "something to help children understand or work out the meaning of more than a single, isolated word" (p 8). In observing the reading period of 24 fourth-grade classrooms for 4,469 minutes, Durkin reported that teachers devoted only *28* minutes (less than 1% of the reading period) to comprehension instruction. Additional observations made during the social studies period (totaling 2,275 minutes) revealed *no* instances of comprehension instruction.

Overtization strategy

Why is there so little "how to" instruction in reading comprehension? One explanation is that the comprehension process is not directly observable, thus making the steps involved in the process difficult to identify, let alone teach. Carnine, Becker, Engelmann, and Kameenui, (1980) conceptualized comprehension skills as cognitive routines involving a series of covert steps, in contrast to physical action routines (such as forming a

Why is there so little "how to" instruction in reading comprehension?

30

letter) involving a series of overt response segments. They proposed that effective teaching of covert routines requires them to be treated as though they were overt physical actions. To do this the teacher must make the usually unobservable steps into overt ones. The advantage of this "overtization" strategy is that teachers can ascertain that learners follow each step and ensure that they are provided feedback on all steps of the routine. Once the learners can perform the steps consistently, producing the desired outcome, they are encouraged to again covertize the process.

Kameenui, Carnine, and Maggs (1980) successfully used an overtized instructional strategy to teach comprehension of reversible passive sentence constructions (e.g., "Sally was teased by Mary"). Carnine et al. (1980, p. 24) described the instructional strategy of overtizing a covert cognitive routine used in that study:

Overt instruction involved initially teaching students to break the complex syntactic construction into two simple sentences. Subsequently, covert self-verbalizations that allowed the children to simplify complex syntactic constructions on their own were taught.

In providing overt instruction for simplifying a passive voice construction, the teacher first verbally modeled the procedure: "Listen, I'll read a sentence and you follow along: Sally was teased by Mary. I can say the sentence another way. Listen, Mary teased Sally. . . ." The learner is then required to apply the strategy with prompting from the teacher: "I'll say the sentence again. 'Sally was teased by Mary.' Now you say the sentence the other way." (Learner: "Mary teased Sally."). The

problem solving strategy shifts from an overtized strategy to covertized strategy when the teacher requires the learner to self-verbalize the strategy: "Now I'm going to say a sentence and ask you a question. Listen, Sally was teased by Mary. Now say it the other way to yourself." Then the teacher asks, "Who did the teasing?" (Learner: "Mary.") "Who got teased? (Learner: "Sally.") After sufficient practice the teacher then utilizes only the convertized strategy and requires the learner to answer novel test questions of a passive voice construction by simply employing the self-verbalization part of the strategy: "Here's a new sentence. . . . Say it the other way to yourself." Complete covertization occurs when the learner answers several items without any teacher prompting.

Direct instruction procedures using the overtization strategy have been applied to several other comprehension skills. In one study, Patching, Kameenui, Colvin, and Carnine (1979) taught students to analyze arguments so as not to be taken in by (a) false causality (just because two things happen around the same time does not mean that one thing causes the other thing); (b) faulty generalization (just because you know about the part does not mean you know about the whole thing); and (c) invalid testimonials (just because someone important in one area says something is good or bad in another area, you cannot be sure it is true).

Woolfson, Kameenui, and Carnine (1979) also taught students to integrate information in passages to make accurate predictions of outcomes. This entailed identifying problem statements, rule statements relevant to the problem statements, information pertinent to the rule statements, and application of the information to solve the problem (i.e., to make the requested prediction).

Finally, Adams (1980) used overtized direct instruction procedures to teach study skills. In this and the previously mentioned studies the direct instruction procedures were compared with conditions involving practice accompanied by corrective feedback (students were told if they were right or wrong during the practice exercises), and with no instruction or practice conditions. In all instances the groups receiving direct instruction procedures surpassed the corrective feedback and no instruction groups on tests measuring the target skills. These results are noteworthy because the conditions involving practice with corrective feedback used the same examples as the direct instruction treatment and students were informed when they were right or wrong. What the conditions did *not* include was "how to" instructions, or in Carnine et al. (1980) terms, overtization of the cognitive routines.

Overtization strategies may not always be necessary for efficient and effective comprehension instruction. Carnine et al. (1980) speculate that providing extensive practice opportunities with corrective feedback may be sufficient to teach simple (i.e., one-step) comprehension skills, as long as the instructional examples are carefully selected. In support of this claim they cite two studies from their laboratory in which a condition involving practice with corrective feedback produced performance equivalent to an overtized condition, with children in both of these conditions surpassing a noninstructed group. In one of these studies students learned to use context clues to identify unknown words (Coyle, Kameenui, & Carnine, nd); in the other they learned to identify story characters' motives (Clements, Stevens, Kameenui, & Carnine, 1979).

Evaluation of direct instruction

In all of the studies reviewed under the topic of direct instruction, the teachers used carefully selected and sequenced examples; taught from scripted lessons which provided precise teacher directions, questions, and correction procedures; required frequent student responding; provided extensive practice so that students reached a mastery criterion before the task was changed; and usually attempted to overtize the normally covert process of comprehension. Clearly the results of these studies suggest that a direct instruction approach holds substantial promise for teaching reading comprehension. However, the results do not suggest that teachers can easily and effectively begin generating their own direct instruction programs. While teachers may wisely borrow ideas from this approach (e.g., overtizing steps in a comprehension skill), the time required to produce instructional programs like those described would be prohibitive. Teachers who find this approach appealing may wish to examine the *Corrective Reading Program*—Comprehension components A, B, and C (Engelmann, Haddux, Hanner, & Osborn, 1978) because this program is an example of a direct instruction approach to teaching reading comprehension.

Now that a technology is available for effectively teaching specific reading skills, which skills are worth teaching?

Ironically, the success of the direct instruction approach raises an important question for which curriculum developers, teachers, reading educators, and reading researchers have yet to provide a satisfactory answer. Specifically, now that a technology is available for effectively teaching specific reading skills, which skills are worth teaching? Certainly some "skills" would not be worth the time and effort because they are rarely needed and because their contribution to comprehension is minimal.

A COGNITIVE PSYCHOLOGY VIEWPOINT

Early behavioral research on reading comprehension focused primarily on procedures that assumed that students were already capable of comprehension (for example, reinforcement for correct answers). More recently curriculum developers have applied behavioral technology in designing programs to *help* students comprehend text. Behavioral researchers have generally used a "bottom-up" analysis of comprehension, emphasizing passage-related skills needed for simplifying complex text (e.g., teaching children how to simplify syntactical patterns). Such bottom-up analyses place less emphasis on the contribution that the reader must make to derive meaning from written material.

Importance of context

Recent research in cognitive psychology suggests that an important determinant of comprehension is the ability of the reader to create a relevant context for interpreting the author's message. The reader's knowledge frameworks or mental schemata interact with the textual cues to create meaning for a given passage. A study by Bransford and Johnson (1972) illustrates the effect of context on the comprehensibility of text. People have difficulty understanding the following passage, even though the vocabulary and syntax are relatively simple.

If the balloons popped the sound wouldn't be able to carry since everything would be too far away from the correct floor. A closed window would also prevent the sound from carrying, since most buildings tend to be well insulated. Since the whole operation depends on a steady flow of electricity, a break in the middle of the wire would also cause problems. Of course, the fellow could shout, but the human voice is not loud enough to carry that far. An additional problem is that a string could break on the instrument. Then there could be no accompaniment to the message. It is clear that the best situation would involve less distance. Then there would be fewer potential problems. With face to face contact, the least number of things could go wrong.

That the absence of an explanatory context is responsible for the incomprehensibility of this passage becomes evident by examining the sketch shown in Figure 1. It is easy to understand why large differences in comprehension are observed between individuals who read this passage with and without the benefit of having seen the "Modern Day Romeo" sketch. These comprehension differences

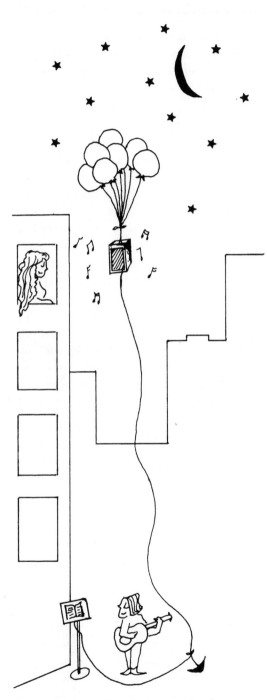

Fig. 1. Modern day Romeo sketch.

33

cannot be explained by arguing that the sketch presents the passage information more clearly, or that it duplicates or contains information expressed in the text. It does neither. Rather, the sketch provides a relevant framework for interpreting the information contained in the text. This simple experiment demonstrates the importance of a relevant framework or background information in the comprehension process.

To make their point Bransford and Johnson composed a reading passage that is admittedly contrived. However, a similar phenomenon can be observed, although to a somewhat lesser degree, in the following passage which was written to approximate those that children are asked to read.

"Goin' Swimming." Part 1.

John swallowed the last drops of orange juice and looked at the sky. He turned to his Dad and said "Dad, will you take Sue and me swimming today?"

Mr. Singer started to answer, then paused. After a moment, he replied "I'd find that enjoyable myself. But first, I better keep my promise about today's yard work."

John bounded up from the table with such enthusiasm that he nearly upset it. Starting toward the garage he shouted "I'll begin collecting the tools now so we can get started."

Now consider the following questions about the events described in the passage.

What is the time of day?
What is the weather like?
What is the meal?
What day of the week?
What season of the year?
Who is Sue?

34

Whom had he promised?
How old is John?
Would they go swimming?
Where would they swim?
In whose yard would they work?
What is Mr. Singer's occupation?

Middle-class adults to whom this task was given tended to respond as follows: The time of day is morning; the day is sunny and warm; the meal is breakfast; it is a weekend; the season is summer; Sue is John's sister; the promise is to Mrs. Singer; John is between 7 and 12 years old; they did decide to go swimming; this event would probably occur at a city pool or possibly a lake; the yard work would occur at home; and Mr. Singer's occupation is unknown.

Importance of background information

Remarkably, none of this information is stated explicitly in the passage, demonstrating how the mental picture that readers constructed went far beyond the information in the text. The richness of this construction results from cognitive contributions generated from the readers' background knowledge or schemata. In this sense, comprehension appears to be a constructive rather than a receptive process.

A text such as this can present comprehension problems for many children, even though they may possess adequate decoding, syntactic, and semantic analysis skills. However, children may not comprehend, because they lack the background knowledge assumed by the writer. For example, in many households children do not develop "breakfast" schemata that include orange juice, "family" schemata

Comprehension and memory for text can be undermined whenever readers lack the background knowledge that would enable them to explain its contents coherently.

that include fathers, "home" schemata that include yards, and "recreation" schemata that include public swimming pools. Children who lack these middle-class, suburban schemata may not generate the interpretation and construction generated by middle-class adults. Not only will the interpretation suffer, but memory too will almost certainly be affected—text that permits the construction of a coherent, understandable, detailed picture is more likely to be remembered than that which prompts the generation of a sketchy impoverished one. Thus comprehension and memory for text can be undermined whenever readers lack the background knowledge that would enable them to explain its contents coherently. In most cases, this is not an all-or-none matter (a notable exception being the Modern Day Romeo selection). More often, individuals probably vary in the number of schemata they own and from which they can create a concrete representation for the "cryptic recipe" that is text (Anderson, 1978).

This conceptualization of reading comprehension permits a description of good comprehenders as individuals who possess numerous and appropriate schemata relevant to a given reading passage, and poor comprehenders as those individuals who lack those schemata altogether or have fewer of them. Comprehension may be viewed as situational—defined in relation to particular reading materials rather than in terms of an enduring trait manifested in all reading situations. This definition of comprehension could explain why children who are generally characterized as poor readers appear to comprehend certain text as well as their classmates who are usually characterized as good readers; on certain passages, at least, the two reader groups possess equivalent sets of background knowledge.

However, it does not explain why children can be classified as good and poor comprehenders in a reliable manner across a variety of reading tests and across a number of reading selections. To accomplish this classification reliably implies that reading comprehension is a general trait rather than one which is situation (text) specific. However, even here a schema explanation is possible. Books pertinent to any specific topic, ranging from astronomy to zoology, are more likely to be found in the Library of Congress than in the Magnolia Branch of the Seattle Public Library. Likewise, individual children differ in the size of their mental libraries as is evident from their performance on instruments such as the WISC information subtest. It follows then that children who own larger, well-stocked libraries will probably have more relevant schemata to apply to diverse reading selections than children whose libraries are small.

Interaction of old and new information

Many children acquire competence in decoding and syntax, yet still differ in their ability to comprehend. These remaining comprehension differences are probably not due merely to *quantitative*

differences in background knowledge. There are several other areas where schema-related breakdowns could impair the ability to comprehend. The following passage, actually the continuation of the "Goin' Swimming" passage, illustrates a schema *utilization* requirement that might create problems for some readers.

"Goin' Swimming." Part 2.

John loaded the rake, clippers, lawn mower and sacks into the back of the truck. Mr. Singer emerged with his appointment book, found the entry that said "Smiths, 101 Cleveland, 1:00 pm, Wednesday."

Climbing in next to John, Mr. Singer said, "It's just over a couple of blocks. If we hurry, we can be there on time."

John turned the key and checked the rear view mirror. Just then, Mr. Singer shouted "Wait, we forgot Sue." He jumped out and gave a loud whistle. In a moment, there was Sue, tearing around the corner of the house. She leapt into the back of the truck and began licking the rear window.

Mr. Singer looked at John and chuckled. "I hope Sue won't mind waiting for her swim until we finish the job."

This second segment of "Goin' Swimming" requires serious modifications of the interpretations suggested by the introductory segment. Actually, the time of day is around noon; the meal is lunch; the day of the week is not Saturday but Wednesday; Sue is a dog, so they probably will not swim in a public pool; the promise was to the Smiths so the yard is at the Smith house; John is old enough to drive; and Mr. Singer's occupation may be gardening. Again it is important to note that the text provides none of this information directly. Instead the reader must revise previous constructions by using

36

new schemata invoked by cues in the text. Apparently the readers' constructions undergo continuous changes as the text provides new data which interact with the previous constructions and with established knowledge structures. This passage illustrates the complex set of relationships among the text, the reader's knowledge, and the representation created from the two.

The process probably operates in the following way. First, readers derive cues from the text, search and select relevant abstract schemata from storage, and apply these schemata to the textual cues to create a concrete formulation that provides meaning. Readers then test the tentative formulation against subsequent textual cues. Based on these tests, readers refine and elaborate, or if necessary discard the previous formulation, and shift to new schemata to derive an altered representation that encompasses all the textual data. While this description of the comprehension process is hypothetical, it would be hard to dispute the claim that individuals who fail to recognize that they have developed an incorrect or inadeqate interpretation for a reading passage, or who have difficulty surrendering an original but incorrect interpretation, will experience comprehension problems.

In addition to comprehension failures that emanate from inadequate world knowledge or rigid adherence to an incorrect construction, deficits may also result when individuals fail to access relevant schemata which they already possess. There is evidence that some learning disabled children possess adequate background knowledge, but do not spontaneously connect textual information with their existing knowledge structures. Wong (1980) developed a memory task, using sentences such as "The boy fell down" that have an implied consequence ("and skinned his knee"). Some sentences were presented with their implied consequence stated (Type I sentences) and others without (Type II sentences). Later, Wong provided the children with recall cues based on the implied consequences. Learning disabled youngsters were able to recall the Type I sentences (with stated consequences) as well as their nonhandicapped peers, but they were less successful on the Type II sentences. This finding is generally taken as evidence that good and poor readers differ in the degree to which they spontaneously elaborate language input. The conclusion that poor readers possess the background knowledge but fail to use it is based on the finding that their recall improved markedly when they were prompted (through a questioning procedure) to elaborate the Type I sentences.

Although this research used an artificial task, recalling sets of unrelated sentences, the findings are nevertheless of potential significance in understanding one problem of poor comprehenders. Certain children apparently possess relevant schemata, but fail to automatically access them perhaps because their threshold for inferring is high (requiring stronger prompts), or because they are satisfied with unelaborated and less detailed representations. Whatever the explanation, good comprehension appears to require a certain amount of active mental processing, and students who do not spontaneously engage in this work are likely to suffer unsatisfactory reading outcomes.

OVERCOMING SCHEMA-RELATED COMPREHENSION PROBLEMS

The conceptualization of reading comprehension as basically a receptive, "bottom-up" process does not work. Experiments from cognitive psychology demonstrate that readers do far more than encode textual information as though the message could stand by itself. Rather, the comprehension process includes a significant "top-down" element wherein readers impose their schemata on the data provided from the text. A more legitimate conceptualization of comprehension recognizes the two-way interaction between existing knowledge and language inputs.

While cognitive psychologists have helped alert students of reading to the role of existing knowledge in the comprehension process, they have not yet translated schema theory into a workable model for instruction. It is one thing to know that children must draw on abstract schemata to formulate concrete representations which are capable of assimilating textual data, but it is another thing to apply this knowledge to instructional practice. However, some general tentative implications for instruction can be derived from schema theory. None of the following instructional proposals have been carefully operationalized, nor thoroughly tested; thus they should be regarded as tentative.

Schema availability

The first proposal addresses the problem of schema availability. We suspect a major variable determining whether individuals will comprehend and remember a specific communication is their background knowledge relevant to the topic of that communication. Indeed, we have gone so far as to speculate that many children who are characterized as poor comprehenders earn this distinction because they lack the requisite background knowledge that authors assume they possess.

If this analysis is accurate, it would seem to indicate an intervention strategy involving a comprehensive and systematic effort to reduce children's knowledge deficits. Most elementary school curriculum plans strongly favor instruction in "tool skills," giving very low priority to the quality of instruction in content areas—with the idea that content instruction can wait until basic skills have been attained. But maybe it cannot. Schools may need to seriously upgrade their content instruction in such areas as the physical, biological, and social sciences so that students are not merely exposed to the concepts, principles, and facts that compose these subject matters, but actually learn them.

This viewpoint is reminiscent of the curriculum revolution of the 1960s, but there is an important difference. While Bruner (1966) and others rightly argued that good content instruction required well-designed curricula which directed students to the important concepts and principles (structure) of a subject matter, they unfortunately tied their proposal to an inefficient and uneconomical instructional format, "discovery learning." A commitment to content instruction does not imply use of a discovery learning model. Direct instruction principles can be applied successfully to the teaching of

38   subject matter so that students acquire basic information and remember it.

An excellent example of effective content instruction, covering such topics as animal taxonomies, body systems, physiology (e.g., skeletal, muscular, and digestive systems), and economics can be seen in the comprehension component of the *Corrective Reading Program* (Engelmann et al., 1978). Concepts and principles have been carefully selected, instructional language and procedures are straightforward and clear, students are brought to criterion on the information taught, they are shown how to apply the information in predicting and explaining events, and the information is frequently reviewed to ensure retention. The contrast between this kind of teaching and that typically found in content curricula is overwhelming. The dismal level of "content" curricula has been documented by Anderson, Armbruster, and Kantor (1980). It is a surprise that students learn anything (if they do) from many of the texts they encounter. At any rate, part of the solution to the reading comprehension problem may reside outside of what is normally considered to be reading instruction.

Active elaboration

While it would be tempting and certainly comforting to assign responsibility for remedying reading comprehension problems to those who design and deliver content instruction, it would not be fair. Not all reading comprehension problems stem from deficits in world knowledge. For example, some students have not learned to adequately use the world knowledge in their possession when given a reading task. They may not spontaneously elaborate text or they may fail to connect the information derived from text with previously acquired relevant schemata.

Addressing this problem, Hanson and Pearson (1980) designed lessons intended to encourage children to elaborate text as they read, thereby enriching the representation which they generated. The lessons consisted of supplying children with "a steady diet of inference" questions during reading. The test of this procedure was to determine if children would better comprehend new passages after having engaged in regular inferencing practice. Hanson and Pearson's results suggested that children given intensive inferencing practice transferred this skill to new passages, because this group outperformed students who had received the regular mix of literal and inference questions (heavily weighted toward the former) prescribed in the teacher's manual. In related studies (Doctorow, 1974; Marks, 1974), investigators obtained comprehension improvements when they required children to restate an idea from each paragraph of a long passage. Doctorow and Marks interpreted these findings as evidence that active elaboration during reading enhances comprehension. Taken together these studies suggest that children can be induced to process text more actively, which in turn may earn them significant dividends in comprehension.

Need to shift schema

The final instructional strategy addresses the schema-related problem that was illustrated in the second segment of the "Goin Swimming" passage: the need for readers to shift schemata when they encounter information that is inconsistent or irreconcilable with a previously developed understanding. We have argued that good readers actively impose abstract schemata onto textual information to create a coherent representation of the author's message. Because good readers are readily inclined to interpret the passage data in terms of their existing knowledge, they place themselves at risk for erroneously interpreting or mistakenly representing the author's meaning based on insufficient information. When this occurs, good readers surrender their original interpretation and seek out an alternative one capable of encompassing all of the passage data. Some poor readers may distinguish themselves from good readers because they are too tolerant of inconsistencies.

The instructional implications, then, would seem to involve helping poor readers, first, to recognize inconsistencies between their formulation and the textual data, and second, to revise their formulation so that it explains all the information in the text. The first problem, recognizing that an interpretation is not consistent with all of the data, is a special case of what Brown (1980) has called "meta-comprehension"—knowing when and what you know, and when and what you do not, and in the latter case knowing what to do about it.

There have been no empirically based attempts to develop procedures for assisting readers to recognize when and what they know. However, good readers engage in regular episodes of self-interrogation during reading. They ask themselves: "Have I been paying attention?" "Do I understand this?" "Could I repeat this?" "Where is all of this leading?" Good readers are also capable of rectifying comprehension or attentional breakdowns by resorting to such strategies as rereading, slowing down, looking back and looking ahead, referring to a table of contents or outline, or seeking outside help (e.g., from a dictionary or an informed source). Possible instructional interventions for students who are unskilled in meta-comprehension strategies may include simple modeling, prompting, and requiring self-interrogatory behaviors during reading. A second set of interventions may involve directly teaching selected fix-up strategies (e.g., rereading) to students who do not use them spontaneously.

• • •

Research on reading comprehension from behavioral and cognitive psychology has tended to emphasize different aspects of comprehension. The former has been more concerned with motivational interventions and specific skill instruction while the latter has emphasized the contribution of the readers' background knowledge. All three aspects—motivation, specific skills, and background knowledge—are important, and with some creativity they can be tapped as sources of interventions for problem readers.

40 REFERENCES

Adams, A.J. The use of direct instruction to teach an independent study method to skill deficient fifth grade students. Unpublished doctoral dissertation, University of Oregon, 1980.

Anderson, R.C. The notion of schemata and the educational enterprise. In R.C. Anderson, R.J. Spiro, & W.E. Montague (Eds.), *Schooling and the acquisition of knowledge*. Hillsdale, N.J.: Lawrence Erlbaum and Associates, 1978.

Anderson, T., Armbruster, B., & Kantor, R.N. How clearly written are children's textbooks; or, of bladderworts and alpha. (Reading Education Report, No. 16.) Urbana: University of Illinois, Center for the Study of Reading, 1980.

Becker, W.L., & Engelmann, S. The direct instruction model. In R. Rhine (Ed.), *Encouraging change in America's schools: A decade of experimentation*. New York: Academic Press, 1977.

Brainerd, C.J. Learning research and Piagetian theory. In L.S. Siegal & C.J. Brainerd (Eds.), *Alternatives to Piaget*. New York: Academic Press, 1977.

Bransford, J.D., & Johnson, M.K. Contextual prerequisites for understanding: Some investigations of comprehension and recall. *Journal of Verbal Learning and Verbal Behavior*, 1972, *11*, 717–726.

Brown, A. Metacognitive development and reading. In R. Spiro, B. Bruce, & W. Brewer (Eds.), *Theoretical issues in reading comprehension*. Hillsdale, N.J.: Lawrence Erlbaum and Associates, 1980.

Bruner, J.S. *Toward a theory of instruction*. Cambridge, Mass.: Harvard University Press, 1966.

Camp, B.W., & Van Doorninck, W.J. Assessment of "motivated" reading therapy with elementary children. *Behavior Therapy*, 1971, *2*, 214–222.

Carnine, D., Becker, W.C., Engelmann, S., & Kameenui, E.J. *Direct instruction analysis of reading*. Unpublished manuscript. Eugene, Ore.: University of Oregon, 1980.

Chall, J. *Learning to read: The great debate*. New York: McGraw-Hill, 1967.

Clements, J., Stevens, C.W., Kameenui, E.J., & Carnine, D.W. Instructional procedures for identifying and interpreting characters' motives during narrative reading. Unpublished manuscript. Eugene, Ore.: University of Oregon, 1979.

Coyle, G., Kameenui, E.J., & Carnine, D.W. A direct instruction approach to teaching the utilization of contextual information in determining the meaning of an unknown word embedded in a passage. Unpublished manuscript. Eugene, Ore.: University of Oregon, undated.

Dahl, P. An experimental program for teaching high speed word recognition and comprehension skills. Final report. Project #3-1154. Washington, D.C.: National Institute of Education, 1974.

Doctorow, M.J. Generative processes in reading. Unpublished doctoral dissertation. University of California at Los Angeles, 1974.

Durkin, D. What classroom observations reveal about reading comprehension instruction. *Reading Research Quarterly*, 1978–1979, *4*, 481–533.

Engelmann, S., Haddux, P., Hanner, S., & Osborn, J. *Thinking basics: Corrective reading program comprehension A*. Chicago: Science Research Associates, 1978.

Engelmann, S., & Steely, D. Final report—Implementation of basal reading in grades 4–6. Unpublished manuscript, 1980.

Fleisher, L.S., Jenkins, J.R., & Pany, D. Effects on poor readers' comprehension of training in rapid decoding. *Reading Research Quarterly*, 1979, *15*, 30–48.

Hansen, C.L., & Lovitt, T.C. The relationship between question type and mode of reading on the ability to comprehend. *Journal of Special Education*, 1976, *10*, 53–60.

Hanson, J. & Pearson, D.P. The effects of inference training and practice on young children's comprehension. (Technical Report No. 166). Urbana: University of Illinois, Center for the Study of Reading, 1980.

Huey, E.B. *The psychology and pedagogy of reading*. New York: Macmillan, 1908.

Jenkins, J.R., Barksdale, A., & Clinton, L. Improving oral reading and comprehension. *Journal of Learning Disabilities*, 1978, *II*, 607–617.

Jenkins, J.R., Pany, D., & Schreck, J. Vocabulary and reading comprehension. (Technical Report No. 100) Urbana: University of Illinois, Center for the Study of Reading, 1978.

Kameenui, E.J., Carnine, D.W., & Maggs, A. Task analysis of instructional procedures for reversible passive and clause constructions. *Exceptional Children*, 1980, *27*, 29–40.

Lahey, B.B., McNees, M.P., & Brown, C.C. Modification of deficits in reading for comprehension. *Journal of Applied Behavior Analysis*, 1973, *6*, 475–480.

Lovitt, T., & Hansen, C. The use of contingent skipping and drilling to improve oral reading and comprehension. *Journal of Learning Disabilities*, 1976, *9*, 481–487.

Marks, C.B. Reading comprehension and structural organization. Unpublished doctoral dissertation, University of California at Los Angeles, 1974.

Pany, D. The effects of vocabulary instruction on knowledge of word meanings and reading comprehension of remedial readers. Unpublished doctoral dissertation, University of Illinois, 1978.

Pany, D., & Jenkins, J.R. Learning word meanings: A comparison of instructional procedures and effects on measures of reading comprehension with learning disabled students. *Learning Disabilities Quarterly*, 1978, *1*, 21–32.

Patching, W., Kameenui, E., Colvin, G., & Carnine, D. An investigation of the effect of using direct instruction procedures to teach three critical reading skills to skill deficient grade 5 children. Unpublished manuscript. Eugene, Ore.: University of Oregon, 1979.

Roberts, M., & Smith, D.D. The relationship among correct and oral reading rates and comprehension. *Learning Disabilities Quarterly*, 1980, *3*, 54–65.

Staats, A.W., & Butterfield, W.H. Treatment of non-reading in a culturally deprived juvenile delinquent: An application of reinforcement principles. *Child Development*, 1965, *36*, 842–925.

Staats, A.W., Minke, K.A., Goodwin, W., & Landeen, J. Cognitive behavior modification: "Motivated learning" reading treatment with subprofessional therapy-technicians. *Behavior Research and Therapy*, 1967, *5*, 283–299.

Wong, B. Activating the inactive learner: Use of questions/prompts to enhance comprehension and retention of implied information in learning disabled children. *Learning Disabilities Quarterly*, 1980, *3*, 29–37.

Woolfson, N., Kameenui, E.J., & Carnine, D.W. Direct instruction procedures for making inferences with variations in the explicitness, complexity, and dispersal of information—An experimental study. Unpublished manuscript. Eugene, Ore.: University of Oregon, 1979.

41

The Route to Reading: A Perspective

Diane J. Sawyer, Ph.D.
Director of Clinical Services
Reading Clinic
Reading and Language Arts Center
Syracuse University
Syracuse, New York

Sally Lipa, Ph.D.
Assistant Professor of Education
State University of New York at Geneseo
Geneseo, New York

DESCRIPTIONS OF THE reading process tend to focus on the competencies that guide readers' interaction with print (Goodman & Niles, 1970) or on the cognitive and linguistic processes that are the substance of those interactions (LaBerge & Samuels, 1974). Currently, no model of reading specifically describes reading behavior within a developmental context that considers what readers bring to the task of learning to read. Nor is there a model that considers how the developmental context affects reading proficiency. A model is needed to facilitate reading instruction that recognizes the possible sources of individual variation in reading behavior. Such a model of reading might also focus research on the interactions among heredity, environment, and learning.

Structure, function, and process capabilities are necessary components of reading behavior. *Structure* refers to the physical network that is responsible for specific kinds of tasks. *Function* is the

0271-8294/81/0012-0043$2.00
© 1981 Aspen Systems Corporation

44

performance capabilities of the physical structures. For example, the brain consists of a variety of separate structures, each one functioning or capable of performing in a specific way and for a specific purpose. *Process* is the application of functional capabilities to the accomplishment of a task. It is initiated outside the structure and function capabilities but must use functional capacity to achieve a product that may be defined as a behavior.

THE ROOTS OF READING BEHAVIOR

Definition of reading

Reading may be broadly defined as the ability to respond to printed language. Responding to language, whether spoken or written, is a communication process. Language is the link between an individual who generates a message and an individual who responds. Language bridges the knowledge base in memory between senders and receivers of messages. The bridge permits meaning to be shared.

Language, whether written or spoken, is a social phenomenon. It functions in a social context and its meaning is rooted in the values, beliefs, traditions, lore, and attitudes of the society. To comprehend a language an individual must be familiar

---

The goal of reading is to construct, out of memory and understanding, personal impressions of the meaning intended by the author.

---

with these and other aspects of the society. The goal of reading is to construct, out of memory and understanding, personal impressions of the meaning intended by the author. These impressions must be sufficiently close to what the author intended to convey for a communication link to be established.

Model of reading behavior

Reading is a process of obtaining meaning; reading comprehension is a subprocess directed toward reconstructing the message within a text. However, getting from print to meaning requires that the reader engage other subprocesses that use auditory and visual perceptual abilities, cognitive (thinking and organizing abilities), language knowledge, and past experiences. Application of these capabilities is dominated by the level of language use growing out of experiences in the sociocultural environment. Thus reading behavior can be viewed as a product of the reader's various perceptual and cognitive ability levels, linguistic ability, expectations regarding interactions in society, and mastery of specific reading task demands (skills). All contribute to the observable levels of reading proficiency. Reading behavior reflects the structure and function of the support system available to a given reader as well as the knowledge base that guides decision making within the system. Figure 1 presents a model of how the major elements of the support system for reading behavior interact. Each element contributes to the development of other elements, and collectively they contribute to the reading process and therefore to reading behavior.

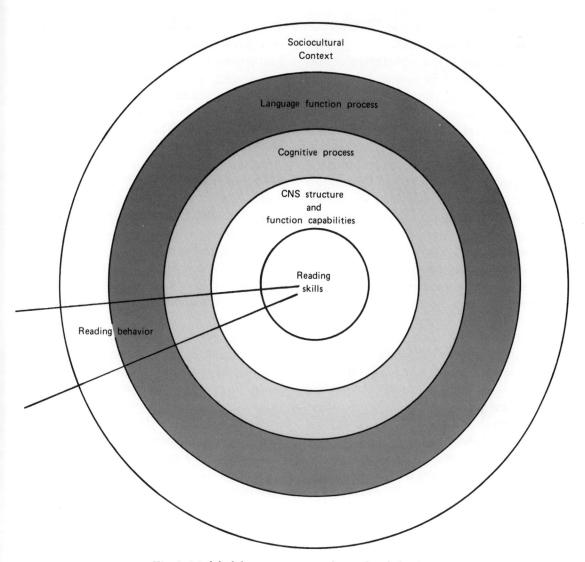

Sociocultural
Context

Language function process

Cognitive process

CNS structure
and
function capabilities

Reading
skills

Reading behavior

Fig. 1. Model of the support system for reading behavior.

Reading skills

The model of the support system for reading behavior shows reading skills, and by implication reading instruction, as the smallest and most embedded support element for reading behavior. Little in the literature on reading instruction suggests that the numerous decoding skills or rules for word analysis and pronunciation are applied by proficient readers. Yet data on disabled readers indicate that limited ability to modify reading behavior following reading instruction is related to central process differences, specific cognitive dys-

46 function, limited linguistic abilities, or specific background factors.

Reading may begin with the print and reading-specific skills taught in reading classes. However, the level of reading competence demonstrated at any given point along the reading continuum is inextricably bound to states of knowledge and information processing capabilities within the various elements of the support system. Reading requires that the reader purposefully engage and coordinate knowledge and competencies available within each element of the support system. Observable reading behavior is an index of what is available and how it is being coordinated across the system.

The interactive view of reading proficiency presented in Figure 1 and the derivable themes developed throughout the remainder of this article are offered to promote an understanding of reading achievement and reading failure. Reading proficiency is a product of biological capabilities and language facility shaped by cultural demands and developed within a social context. This base for perceptual, cognitive, and linguistic function is available for activation and subsequent shaping during reading instruction at school. Kleinfeld's (1973) discussion of the intellectual strengths among culturally different groups showed the nature of these concepts of "interaction" and "product."

Sociocultural context

Kleinfeld (1973) used Eskimos as an example to demonstrate that different cognitive strengths may be identified among culturally different groups. This is a consequence of the ecological demands made by a particular environment. Kleinfeld argued that the group's cultural adaptations to these demands stimulated the development of particular types of cognitive abilities. Specifically, Eskimos hunt in the Arctic terrain, which is visually uniform. These hunters must be exceptionally sensitive to the most minute visual detail to ensure safety on the ice, to judge impending weather changes, and to find the way back home. Awareness of figural detail and the ability to memorize such detail are critical to successful movement through the Arctic.

Kleinfeld described how the Eskimo language reflects the cultural adaptation to the environment. Its structure seems uniquely suited to aid the processing of figural information. In Eskimo it is obligatory to specify both the shape of the object and the shape of the surface on which it is placed (possible by adding prefixes and suffixes). Three-word sentences may be used to convey all this information in Eskimo, while several more words would be required in English. "Because localizers permit economical coding of spatial information, the speaker of the Eskimo language may also find such information easier to remember than speakers of English" (p. 345).

Kleinfeld continued by showing how childrearing practices that foster exploration, social exchanges such as lengthy storytelling sessions focused on detailing physical features of specific terrain observed (i.e., a fork in a river), and the gene pool (as it represents the characteristics of those who were capable of adapting to the demands of the environment and thus of surviving) contribute to the development of high-level figural abilities among the Eskimos. These abilities are critical to survival in the Arctic, just as verbal skills, especially reading, are critical to economic survival in a technological society. But figural abilities apparently have little value in the Western-oriented schools Eskimos attend, where they generally achieve little success. However, Tough (1977) suggested that even within Western societies the values of subcultures structure experiences, interactions, and language. Thus different intellectual strengths emerge and different levels of school success result.

Language and cognitive functions

Sociocultural experiences provide the background for learning. These experiences affect the development of patterns for perceptual and cognitive responses to the environment. As a result, sociocultural experiences determine the extent to which biological capabilities for perceptual and cognitive function will be realized.

The model presented in Figure 1 shows neurophysiological capabilities as embedded within environmental influences and therefore subject to both maturation and learning. Language and cognitive functions are represented as functions that span neurophysiological capabilities and sociocultural experiences. The shading in Figure 1 is to emphasize that these functions develop and are refined as a consequence of interactions during learning between the sociocultural context and the structure and function capabilities of the central nervous system (CNS). The interactive view of the development of linguistic and cognitive function focuses on the role of individual variation in CNS function and differences in environmental

context. Educators are attempting to understand the effect of such variations on the development of linguistic capabilities and on the attainment of the more sophisticated levels of cognitive function necessary for skilled reading.

THE SOCIOCULTURAL FOUNDATION OF LANGUAGE AND READING BEHAVIOR

Differences in language use

Reading is a language activity, and language is learned in a social context. Differences in language use are observable among people of different geographic regions, ethnic groups, social groups, and educational backgrounds. Differences in language behavior develop from social expectations and conventions for the use of language learned along with language. These expectations and conventions concerning language use affect thinking behavior and ultimately reading behavior. A recent longitudinal study, conducted by Tough (1977) in England, permits inference regarding some of the interactions between social context, language use, and patterns of thinking and analyzing at different stages of individual development. The findings suggest a relationship between social class background, language use, and language comprehension, with serious implications for reading achievement and school success.

Tough found that at age 3 differences were noted in the kinds of meanings that were imposed on experiences and expressed through language when advantaged children (from families of professional or semiskilled workers) and disadvantaged children (from families of

48 unskilled workers) were compared. Different sociocultural backgrounds may influence ideas of what aspects of a situation are of primary importance and therefore meaningful.

At age 5½, the disadvantaged group demonstrated a general failure to infer possible relationships, causes, and consequences when they were asked to interpret happenings in pictures. They apparently had difficulty sorting out which information was important and how the bits related. Further, the disadvantaged children found it difficult to project into the future world of "what might be." Their discussions included mainly descriptive labeling and they were inclined to be both less explicit about their ideas and less aware of the range of interpretations possible for the information given. At age 7½, most of these children scored near but below the norm in a measure of reading that required both decoding and comprehension. Tough concluded that "the development and use of language must be seen as the major means through which . . . (educational) . . . objectives . . . may be reached" (p. 173).

Reasons for differences in language use

Modeling

Why do such differences in language use and comprehension arise? Studies of language development and of cognitive development for reasoning over the past 15 years suggest that people learn the language modeled in the home. Such modeling is inherent in the language adults use in interactions with children. Research findings suggest that cultural

Cultural differences yield differences in the vocal-verbal behavior of children, the problem-solving strategies of children, and the reasoning capabilities available within different cultural subgroups.

differences yield differences in the vocal-verbal behavior of children, the problem-solving strategies of children, and the reasoning capabilities available within different cultural subgroups as a consequence of adult verbal interactions with children.

Irwin (1948) studied the amount of vocal productions observed among infants from different cultural backgrounds. The number and frequency of sounds produced were lower among infants age 18 months and beyond who were being reared in low-income homes. In a subsequent study Irwin (1960) found that the vocal productions of such children between the ages of 13 months and 30 months increased when the children were regularly read stories. Presumably, the lower-class infants were not experiencing as much language around them, or directed toward them. Thus they were not as stimulated to produce utterances themselves. Reading stories to children was viewed as one means of increasing the amount of language stimulation a child received.

Value systems

Lesser (1964), in a study of the mental abilities of children from different social classes and cultural groups, found that among Chinese, Jewish, Negro, and Puerto Rican first graders, Jewish children excelled in verbal skills while Chinese children were superior in visual and spatial relationships. This was interpreted as evidence that different cultural subgroups, as a group, possess different values concerning the skills and abilities they foster in their children. While some groups place a high value on skillful use of language and foster these skills, perhaps at the sacrifice of certain other skills, other groups value manual dexterity or physical development over verbal skills. Children develop early those skills which are most emphasized and fostered at home.

Environmental deprivation

Cross-cultural studies have looked at achievement of the levels of logical thought described by Piaget (Dasen, 1972). In many societies many or even most adults do not attain the level of concrete operations that appears at about age 7 in the culture of many Western countries. Even in the United States only about 30% of the adults display thought at the level of formal operations (presumably achieved between age 11 and age 14).

Epstein (1978) suggested that the low levels of logical thought might be caused by environmental deprivation. Personal interactions within a culture cause individuals to develop thinking and reasoning skills required to succeed in that culture. Although the biological potential to learn to reason abstractly may be available, only appropriate experiences in society will permit that potential to be realized.

Tough's findings suggest that even within a Western technological society, children from certain kinds of social contexts do not learn to relate and organize information in ways valued in school.

Schooling

Olson (1977) argued that "schooling, particularly learning to read, is the critical process in the transformation of children's language" (p. 278) from a basic dependence on the *context* in which language is used to convey a part of the message, to the use of language as the primary and even exclusive conveyor of meaning. Olson argued that in a society dominated by written language, "assumptions and premises are made explicit, formal rules of logic are observed, and individuals operate on careful definitions" (p. 278). Reading language that is so structured is seen as a powerful vehicle for shaping the ability to reason carefully and logically. Spoken language will then also reflect those thinking and reasoning strategies and levels of abstraction.

Professionals and skilled workers generally have achieved some level of success during their school years. Thus they have developed the patterns of thinking and reasoning that promote or foster school success. Language use in such families reflects these patterns of thinking and for expressing thought.

However, within some subcultures, school success is not a personal value among many parents. Little, if any, daily reading occurs. Oral language tends to be tied to the setting in which it occurs, and there is great reliance on nonverbal communication. What children learn as

50

they become effective listeners and speakers in that social context is probably not adequate preparation for what must be known about language comprehension and use to interact effectively in the classroom. The "advantage" some families provide their children may not be a range of experiences or varieties of vocabulary labels for the world, but rather a means for using language to describe, organize, and act on the world.

Organization of thought processes

Thorndike (1917) in his discussion of reading, stated that "Reading *is* Reasoning." He proposed that limited comprehension reflects limited thinking and reasoning abilities. Thorndike suggested that poor comprehension may indicate inadequate intellectual processing. For more than 60 years, educators have interpreted consistently low comprehension scores as evidence of limited intelligence.

An examination of the research in various areas of child development suggests another possible interpretation. Studies of the development of perceptual abilities, cognitive organization, and language acquisition suggest instead that poor comprehension may reflect a different organization of the intellectual processes a child applies. Individuals differ in the organization of the thought processes that guide selection of what is important to attend to, how to organize it, and what to say about it. Individual variation in the organization of thought processes is probably rooted in values and organizational patterns. These patterns are modeled in the social context in which the child acquires language and learns to use language for communication.

THE STRUCTURAL AND FUNCTIONAL CAPABILITIES OF THE CENTRAL NERVOUS SYSTEM

The structures of the central nervous system (CNS) are biologically determined. However, the development of the functions associated with these structures is subject to stimulation, support, and modification as a result of experiences encountered within the sociocultural context. Reading behavior must be viewed as evidence of the application of these functions to the reading task.

Reading is a process requiring both perceptual and conceptual tasks. Reading behavior depends on biologically determined structures, capacities for their function, and the efficiency of information processing in the nervous system.

Cerebral cortex

One CNS structure important for reading behavior is the cerebral cortex. The cerebral cortex is composed of two hemispheres, right and left. These hemispheres are connected by bands of fibers called commissures. The largest band of these fibers is the corpus callosum and is considered important in the transmission of information across the hemispheres.

Right hemisphere

The right hemisphere appears to organize and treat data as wholes, "being in effect a synthesizer—of information, viewing the total configuration rather than parts" (Nebes, 1974, p. 3). The right hemisphere treats nonverbal information and stores information as units. These units are spatial or auditory (Kimura,

1966). The right hemisphere organizes information based on structural similarities. Sensory data are reconstructed to form perceptual wholes (Lezak, 1976).

Left hemisphere

In contrast, the left hemisphere sequentially analyzes input and "abstracts out relevant details with which it associates verbal symbols" (Nebes, 1974, p. 4). In most individuals the left hemisphere is the language hemisphere. All verbal transformations of reading, writing, understanding, speaking, verbal ideation, and comprehension of verbal symbols traced on the skin are mediated in the left hemisphere or the language hemisphere of the brain. The left hemisphere organizes information based on conceptual similarities. Tasks such as finding similarities in meaning between bits of information, labeling, and categorization are functions of the left hemisphere (Nebes, 1974).

Within the left hemisphere of the cerebral cortex at least four specific areas serve the processes required for language and reading: Broca's area, Wernicke's area, the visual cortex, and the angular gyrus. Broca's area appears to be primarily responsible for speech and language production. Wernicke's area is primarily responsible for comprehension of speech and language. These areas are connected by a bundle of fibers that allows for the transmission of signals between regions.

The visual cortex lies behind the speech and language areas. This area and the language comprehension area (Wernicke's) are connected by a specialized area, the angular gyrus, which is a "way station" or integration area for both audi-

tory and visual stimuli within the language hemisphere (Geschwind, 1972). Geschwind gives the following example of the transmission of signals in this area during reading. "When a word is read, the output from the primary visual area passes to the Angular Gyrus, which in turn arouses the corresponding auditory form of the word in Wernicke's area" (p. 79). Thus the angular gyrus seems to be necessary for the interaction of visual and auditory information. Injury or developmental dysfunction in this area could lead to reading difficulty.

Information processing

Role of memory

In reading, beyond the integration of visual and auditory stimuli, the brain must also use incoming stimuli so that the information can be organized and take on meaning. An important aspect of information processing is how the brain organizes information between the time it receives it and the time it responds with an output signal.

Information processing involves the transformation of the signals that enter the brain into usable information. This transformation uses both information already stored or known about the world and newly received information. Therefore memory plays an important role in information processing.

Calfee (1975) defines memory as "an interrelated set of psychological processes for encoding, storing and retrieving information. At one end, memory becomes indistinguishable from perception, at the other end it merges with skilled performance" (p. 70). Because reading requires

52

that information be processed from visual perception to conceptual development or refinement, memory is necessary for reading. It pervades the individual components of the reading task—recognizing letters, words, and meanings—by providing lines of communication between and among these discrete elements. Memory is the framework that permits associations to be made and organization to be achieved.

Hemispheric specialization

Developmentally, each hemisphere of the brain achieves specialization of function through a normal maturational process. Early research by Kimura (1963) using dichotic listening tasks suggested that by age 4 language in children has lateralized to the left hemisphere, with girls showing superior lateralization to boys. Lateralization continues to develop in children through age 7. This suggests that many children are being taught to read while hemispheric specialization for language is still developing.

Recent investigations into the role of hemispheric lateralization in reading achievement indicate that lateralization is still incomplete among some first- and second-grade children. Bakker, Tennison, and Bosch (1976) suggested that the beginning level tasks in reading might develop easily before the dominant hemisphere for language has been established. The results suggest that when the reading task requires primarily perceptual, holistic responses to print—as in the acquisition of whole words as sight words—the need for specific language function, which is specific in the left or language hemisphere, is insignificant. But later, when reading requires primarily concep-

tual activity, the need for language function is essential. Witelson (1977) indicated that the poor reader or "dyslexic" may not develop the normal lateralization of function common to most individuals. In addition, poor readers exhibit an overdeveloped use of spatial, holistic functioning. These results suggest the importance of the development of appropriate hemispheric specialization within the maturing child as a support for the attainment of reading proficiency.

The attainment of reading proficiency has also been shown to depend on the ways that the functional capabilities of the central nervous system are individually applied. The recent use of evoked potentials as a measure of brain functioning has disclosed differences in brain electrical activity between normal and disabled readers. The evoked potential technique measures brain electrical activity to some distinct event, such as a light flash or a word. When a stimulus is presented a change in electrical activity can be detected. This change is defined as a response to the stimulus. The responses of disabled readers to evoked potentials tend to suggest some degree of neurological dysfunction. Within this group, more time elapses between presentation of the stimulus and the change in electrical activity recorded. However, delayed response may also suggest immaturity in the central nervous system (Connors, 1969; Preston, Guthrie, & Childs, 1974; Shields, 1973).

In summary, research indicates that reading depends on the development of the CNS and the cerebral cortex, consisting of a right and a left hemisphere. These structures take on the specialized functions necessary for reading. These func-

Reading depends on the development of the central nervous system and the cerebral cortex.

tions involve the receiving and storing as well as the organization, integration, and encoding of auditory and visual stimuli. As the brain matures, function capabilities become hemisphere specific. The left hemisphere becomes dominant for language function while the right becomes dominant for spatial and holistic functions. Lateralization of language appears to be necessary for acquiring proficiency in reading. Individual variations in the application of functional capabilities within the CNS are related to differences in reading performance.

READING PROFICIENCY

Reading proficiency is a function of the various perceptual and cognitive ability levels, social expectations, and reading task demands that contribute to the observable levels of reading achievement. The model of reading presented in Figure 2 is an attempt to describe the developmental progression toward reading mastery. A child in a literate society enters into this progressive, adaptive sequence at birth. The developmental view considers the interplay of environment, heredity, maturation, and learning as they affect progress toward reading proficiency.

Figure 2 illustrates the interaction of the human endowments for linguistic and social interactions, maturation, learning, and the behavior possible as a result of these interactions. This model describes the pathway traveled from development

of the support system that serves reading, through the stage of learning to read, and on to the stage of reading to learn. Within this model, the capabilities for cognitive-linguistic functioning that develop before school entrance serve the "learning-to-read" stage of development. However, they are shaped, modified, and extended as a consequence of the accommodations made within the system. The accommodations are a response to both the mechanical aspects of learning to read (i.e., the requirements for visual and auditory perceptual activity associated with relating printed and spoken language), and the conceptual development and refinement associated with reading as a tool for learning.

Before reading begins

At the moment of conception each individual receives the full complement of potentials that may be realized in the course of a lifetime. Along with the potentials for the maximum achievable height and general intelligence, each person also receives, through the genes, the potentials for learning language and thus for interacting with others. Intrauterine development is affected by maternal health and nutrition as well as genetic endowment. The attainment of innate potentials depends on the nurturing environment from the moment of conception.

At birth a child enters the social environment. The neurophysiological capabilities and potentials for collecting, organizing, and acting on information that have been realized during the prenatal period now engage an environment of objects, people, and states or relationships (hot-cold; near-far). Stimulation from the envi-

54

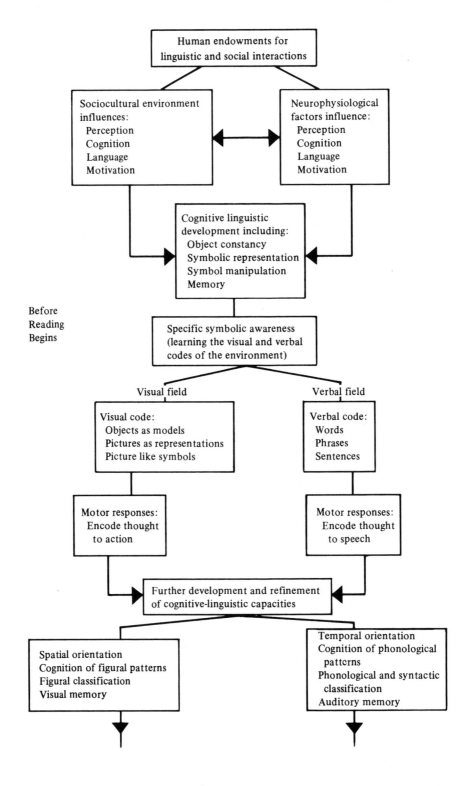

Before
Reading
Begins

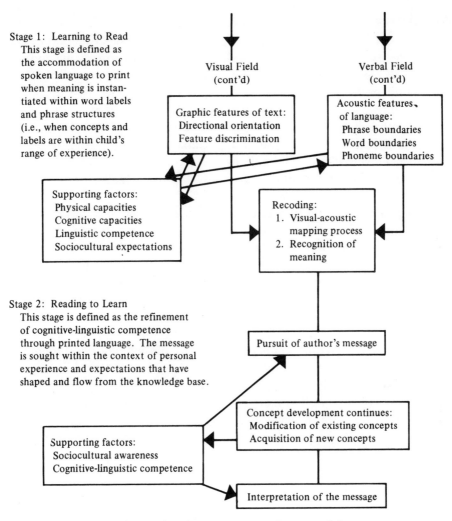

Stage 1: Learning to Read
This stage is defined as the accommodation of spoken language to print when meaning is instantiated within word labels and phrase structures (i.e., when concepts and labels are within child's range of experience).

Visual Field (cont'd)

Verbal Field (cont'd)

Graphic features of text:
Directional orientation
Feature discrimination

Acoustic features of language:
Phrase boundaries
Word boundaries
Phoneme boundaries

Supporting factors:
Physical capacities
Cognitive capacities
Linguistic competence
Sociocultural expectations

Recoding:
1. Visual-acoustic mapping process
2. Recognition of meaning

Stage 2: Reading to Learn
This stage is defined as the refinement of cognitive-linguistic competence through printed language. The message is sought within the context of personal experience and expectations that have shaped and flow from the knowledge base.

Pursuit of author's message

Concept development continues:
Modification of existing concepts
Acquisition of new concepts

Supporting factors:
Sociocultural awareness
Cognitive-linguistic competence

Interpretation of the message

Fig. 2. A developmental view of reading as a cognitive-linguistic ability.

ronment, opportunities to act on the environment, and lessons learned through interactions within the environment stimulate and shape the development of innate perceptual, cognitive, and linguistic capabilities. They also foster levels of curiosity or motivation for seeking experiences in the environment. Neurophysiological capabilities in infancy and childhood control the type and level of interaction with the environment. Children with physical or mental handicaps cannot achieve the same levels of interaction as "normal" children. In turn, the opportunities for experience and learning that are permitted or available within the environment guide and channel the development of cognitive and linguistic abilities during infancy and early childhood.

Figure 2 shows that interactions in the environment during infancy lead to the development of the specific cognitive and

56 linguistic abilities. These abilities support the use of visual and verbal symbols to code the world. The flow diagram shows some of the specific elements that must be mastered within each type of code system. In addition, during early childhood children gain control over motor responses. This makes it possible for children to use action, visual, or verbal code systems to "encode" or represent and communicate thought.

The process of learning the elements of these codes and of learning to use the codes for communication results in further development and refinement of cognitive and linguistic capacities. In the visual field the importance of spatial relationships and orientation of figures on a plane, recognition of patterns of details (details in relation to each other), recognition of common characteristics of different figures (corners, sides, edges, lines, curves, size, and color) as well as memory for visual details and patterns develop. In the verbal field, related development involves recognition of the importance of the order or sequences of sounds and words over time (Sally hit Mary versus Mary hit Sally; top versus pot), recognition of patterns in the spoken language as alliteration, rhyming, phrasing, or emphasis, and organization of speech elements according to common characteristics (as in noting plurals—recognizing when the various forms are appropriate—ducks, tapes versus dogs, toes versus feet, mice). Auditory memory for sounds, names, meaning, and the effects of order on their interpretation also develops significantly during preschool years.

When a child learns to read, the degree of ease and success experienced depends on the level of development achieved in these prerequisite capabilities for recognizing patterns, organizing and classifying information, and interpreting information in terms of knowledge of the structure and function of language. Memory for prior experiences and the connotations of spatial or temporal reorganization of those experiences also contribute significantly to learning to read.

Learning to read

The *learning-to-read stage* is narrowly defined as the time during which children sort out the distinguishing features of print symbols and understand the linkages between printed language and spoken language. In the visual field the specific learning that occurs at this stage centers on discrimination of and memory for the features that distinguish printed letters and words. In the verbal field, many children are simultaneously learning that a spoken message is made up of parts smaller than sentences. Their awareness of spoken language is being refined, and they can independently separate phrases within sentences, individual words that make up a message and, finally, the individual sounds that make up a word.

The level of development and function that has been achieved among the various supporting factors both contributes to this learning process and is modified as a consequence of this learning. Children learn that printed shapes or forms can be linked with particular sounds and word labels. They recognize that the message is bound to the features of the print at one level and to the ideas and experiences that they have stored in memory and can access through words and phrases. Words that might have been thought to have multiple meanings when they were only heard in spoken language come to be understood as different words because of their spelling (meet/meat, would/wood). Elements that may have been understood to form a single unit when heard come to be recognized as discrete as a result of the way they are presented for teaching as well as the size of spaces around them when printed ("lmno" in the alphabet or common phrases such as "inthe," "wanna-go").

During this stage, specific links are forged between the right and left hemispheres of the brain to facilitate "automatic" responses to printed language at the various levels—from saying words to recognizing or associating meaning with the label to recognizing the need for and thus to activate cognitive processes that order or reorder stored or incoming information to derive meaning. Background knowledge, language knowledge, and the functional capabilities of the CNS must all be coordinated for the search-respond-search procedure that characterizes reading. Further, children must learn to direct this procedure sometimes to the page and sometimes to thought processes, and memory as the focus of reading shifts from saying words and "getting meaning" instantly to saying words and trying to "figure out" meaning.

When careful evaluations are conducted, reading difficulties at the learning-to-read stage can often be traced back to deficiencies within the support system for reading. Problems related to mastery at this stage of reading are usually the most serious examples of reading difficulties. They are frequently the most diffi-cult to overcome using the traditional reading skill remediation practices typically employed. Brief sketches of children from the Syracuse University Reading Clinic files show the problems related to factors within the support system. The cases also show the limitations such knowledge and process difficulties impose on the potential for achieving reading success when typical instructional procedures are employed.

Charles, age 12, had not yet mastered naming letters and knew only about 25 high frequency words at sight. He could not generate words that followed a rhyming pattern provided for him. He could spell only two words other than his name. Charles had repeated first grade and had received special, intensive help in reading since first grade. He was bright and verbal, but could not learn to read. He could learn in school through listening and did well on tests when they were read to him, and he could answer orally. Charles' medical history indicated a series of convulsions at the age of 2 weeks, stemming from a severe calcium deficiency during the prenatal period. His developmental history indicated delays in the development of all motor areas. Damage or dysfunction in the CNS (perhaps in the right hemisphere) undoubtedly is related to the extreme difficulty Charles experienced at the learning-to-read stage.

Connie, age 23, a mother, was hoping to improve her reading sufficiently to get and keep a job. She had dropped out of high school and had always done poorly in school. She reported being embarrassed often because she could not consistently say the words she saw on the page. Connie had had speech therapy in elementary school and still had what her tutor described as "strange speech patterns." When she read aloud she frequently would

58

stop to "work out a word." She seemed to recognize many of the words, often could offer related words, but just could not "get out" the appropriate word. An in-depth evaluation of Connie's hearing and auditory processing abilities at a medical center indicated good acuity. Problems discriminating and organizing linguistic information suggested a neurological difficulty. Connie's oral reading behavior and her own descriptions of the problems she had with reading suggest that her difficulties in learning to read probably stem from dysfunction in the language hemisphere (perhaps involving the angular gyrus, as discussed earlier).

Paul, age 10, called words well. Even in the first grade his teacher had been concerned that he did not seem to pay attention to the meaning of what he read. Paul was the youngest of two boys in a close, middle-class family. He loved sports and spent all his out-of-school time swimming, playing baseball, and going to ball games. He did not watch much television, nor did he play cards or board games. Most talk at home and in his circle of friends focused on active sports. At the beginning of fourth grade he demonstrated word recognition abilities that were at grade level but reading comprehension was more consistent with end-of-first-grade competencies. His knowledge of words and overall use of language suggested that Paul was tied to concrete experiences. His full-scale IQ on a WISC test, administered as part of the reading diagnosis, was 64. Clearly the reasoning abilities Paul had available to bring to reading were limited. Undoubtedly, his good word recognition performance, his ability to succeed socially, and the strength of the supportive home environment concealed his cognitive deficiencies during the early primary-grade years when so much instruction time and evaluation are directed toward efficient recoding of printed symbols.

Mary was a shy second grader. She read slowly, haltingly, and without expression. Her responses to questions about her reading were somewhat vague or literal. She had average intelligence and adequate oral language for her age. Mary's family lived on a fairly remote farm and belonged to a strict religious group. Mary had only animal playmates outside of school. Books were considered "tools of the devil" and a letter had been sent to Mary's teacher each year indicating that Mary was not to go to the school library and that no books were to be sent home with Mary. Only the Bible was read at home. Mary had never seen a television program or gone to a movie. Once each week she accompanied her parents to town to buy groceries and other necessities. On Sunday most of the day was spent at church services and in prayer and contemplation.

Mary's difficulties at the learning-to-read stage apparently stemmed from limited experiences in the world as well as a probable fear of reading stemming from the kinds of stories she met in the basic reader that must have seemed "sinful" to Mary's innocent mind. The values, attitudes, and experiences Mary encountered in her home environment had not prepared her to meet the demands of learning to read in school. The instructional materials used in school, as well as the attitudes concerning the purpose for reading that underlie teaching behavior in schools, opposed everything Mary understood to be "truth." Even if Mary did become fluent at recoding, it is doubtful that she would "succeed" in reading. Mary was not encouraged to think critically, to analyze, to balance different bits of information against each other, and to draw conclusions based on information. Mary was "commanded" and taught to "accept" without question. The range of her vocabulary will remain restricted in an environment devoid of books, newspapers, and nonprint media and where contacts with other people are limited. Even experiences provided in and through the school setting are likely to have limited impact until Mary permits herself to be touched by them. Mary will continue to have difficulty recognizing the meaning intended to be cued by printed language.

Reading to learn

During this stage readers use cognitive and linguistic competencies, including specific reading skills, as well as awarenesses about their own and other cultures to actively pursue the message the author intended to convey. The process requires organizing stored information, ideas, experiences, and impressions cued by printed language in an attempt to reconstruct the meaning as the author might have intended. In the process, old information is viewed in new ways, new information is taken in, and this extends or modifies prior concepts. Entirely new concepts also take shape in the process.

The attainment of new concepts or the modification of existing concepts through reading requires the application of cognitive-linguistic competencies to printed language. In turn, this stimulates further development and refinement of those competencies. Evidence of that development and refinement is shown through increased vocabularies, greater ability to understand complex grammatical structures or patterns of paragraph organization, softened prejudices, greater objectivity, and greater facility with abstract concepts. However, the message grasped through reading is always colored by the base of awarenesses and competencies applied to the task of reconstructing the author's message. What is on the page is subject to individual interpretation. Misinterpretation, as well as error, in getting the intended message is therefore possible throughout an individual's reading lifetime.

CONCLUSION

This article has provided an opportunity to pose a perspective on reading, reading difficulties, and reading instruction that highlights the role of child development in reading achievement; to focus attention on those aspects of individual variation that educators must acknowledge as they try to identify, circumvent, and overcome reading difficulties. The models presented are intended to be illustrative rather than definitive. At this time they must be understood as evolving models. But the implications of the perspective expressed through these models for educational practice are clear. The energies devoted to reading instruction, particularly remedial reading instruction, which are typically focused on specific "reading skills," must be balanced against an understanding of the knowledge and process foundations for learning. Successful teaching must be rooted in the knowledge of what each child has available, at the level of knowledge and processing capabilities, to permit learning that which is being taught (even if it is assumed that what is being taught is essential for learning to read).

Identifying the *critical* differences

60

among children at the learning-to-read stage could contribute significantly to increasing reading success. Increasing teacher awareness of the nature, source, and range of individual differences at the learning-to-read stage will undoubtedly serve the end of *early* identification of "at risk" children. But methods for inferring the nature of the difficulty a child is experiencing must be developed. Strate-gies for coping with processing difficul-ties, either for teaching reading or for circumventing reading to promote con-tinued learning, must be explored. Research that can serve these ends must abandon correlational designs that seek to identify the "common denominator" and focus instead on the observable reading behaviors that underscore the nature of individual differences.

REFERENCES

Bakker, D.J., Tennison, J., & Bosch, J. Development of laterality—reading patterns. In R.M. Knights & D.J. Bakker (Eds.), *The neuropsychology of learning disorders: Theoretical approaches*. Baltimore: University Park Press, 1976.

Calfee, R. Memory and cognitive skills in reading acquisition. In D. Duane & M. Lawson (Eds.), *Reading perception and language*. Baltimore: York Press, 1975, 55–95.

Connors, C.R. Auditory synthesis and dichotic listening in children with learning disabilities. *Journal of Special Education*, 1969, 3, 163–170.

Dasen, P.R. Cross-cultural Piagetian research: A summary. *Journal of Cross-Cultural Psychology*, 1972, 3, 23–29.

Epstein, H.T. Growth spurts during brain development: Implications for educational policy and practice. In J.S. Chall & A.F. Mirsky (Eds.), *Education and the brain* (77th yearbook of the National Society for the Study of Education). Chicago: University of Chicago Press, 1978.

Galaburda, A., Le May, M., Kemper, T., & Geschwind, N. Right left asymmetries in the brain. *Science*, 1978, 199, 852–856.

Geschwind, N. Language and the brain. *Scientific American*, 1972, 76–85.

Goodman, K.S., & Niles, O. *Reading processes and product*. Urbana, Ill.: National Council of Teachers of English, 1970.

Irwin, O.C. Infant speech: The effect of family occupational status and of age on sound frequency. *Journal of Speech and Hearing Disorders*, 1948, 13, 320–333.

Irwin, O.C. Infant speech: Effect of systematic reading of stories. *Journal of Speech and Hearing Disorders*, 1960, 3, 187–190.

Kimura, D. Speech lateralization in young children as determined by an auditory test. *Journal of Comparative and Physiological Psychology*, 1963, 56, 899–902.

Kimura, D. Dual function asymmetry of the brain in visual perception. *Neuropsychologia*, 1966, 4, 275–285.

Kleinfeld, J.F. Intellectual strengths in culturally different groups: An Eskimo illustration. *Review of Educational Research*, 1973, 43(3), 341–359.

LaBerge, D., & Samuels, S.J. Toward a theory of automatic information processing in reading. *Cognitive Psychology*, 1974, 6, 293–323.

Lesser, G., Fiefer, G., & Clark, D. Mental abilities of children in different social and cultural groups. *Monograph of the Society for Research in Child Development*, 1964, Report No. CRP–1635.

Lezak, M.D. *Neuropsychological assessment*. New York: Oxford University Press, 1976.

Luria, A. Cerebral organization of conscious acts: A frontal lobe function. In L. Tarnipol & M. Tarnipol (Eds.), *Brain function and reading disabilities*. Baltimore: University Park Press, 1977.

Nebes, R.D. Hemispheric specialization in commissurotomized man. *Psychological Bulletin*, 1974, 81, 1, 1–14.

Olson, D. From utterances to text: The bias of language in speech and writing. *Harvard Educational Review*, 1977, 47(3), 257–281.

Preston, M., Guthrie, J., & Childs, B. Visual evoked responses in normal and disabled readers. *Psychophysiology II*, 1974, 452–457.

Shields, D. Brain responses to stimuli in disorders of information processing. *Journal of Learning Disability*, 1973, 6, 501–505.

Thorndike, E.L. Reading as reasoning. *Journal of Educational Psychology*, 1917, 8, 323–332.

Tough, J. *The development of meaning*. New York: John Wiley & Sons, 1977.

Witelson, S. Developmental dyslexia: Two right hemispheres and none left. *Science*, 1977, 309–311.

Child Reading: Readiness or Evolution?

D. Kim Reid, Ph.D.
Assistant Professor
University of Texas
Dallas, Texas

JUST PRIOR to the turn of the century, when free, public schooling began to be taken seriously as a national responsibility and total literacy became a national goal, educators and psychologists discovered that many children were not learning to read and many more were experiencing great difficulty. The search for possible explanations resulted in the educational application of the concept of readiness. The concept of readiness does not, however, represent a single explanation for reading problems. It represents three explanations: maturation, experience, and task-ability matches. To explain the changing nature of the concept of readiness and to explicate a fourth position (which I shall refer to as the evolution of child reading), a discussion of each orientation is necessary. The presentation of the first three positions will be brief. The interested reader is encouraged to read Durkin's (1968) comprehensive review of the early literature, which includes an overview of the development

0271-8294/81/0012-0061$2.00

62 of the first two positions and articulates the third—a position Durkin was largely responsible for popularizing. The evolution of the child reading model, or rather emerging trends within that model, will constitute the major thrust of this discussion. My purpose is to suggest that children's reading begins gradually and evolves spontaneously during the preschool years. Consequently, the concept of readiness in its traditional senses is superfluous.

CONCEPTS OF READINESS

Several of the earliest workers to study readiness viewed it as a maturational phenomenon. A counter group, formed as the maturationist position became clearly articulated, emphasized the early environmental experiences of children. Their focus was on the development of enabling capacities that would permit children to begin to read. A third position, not widely acceptable until the 1960s, suggested that the key to children's readiness for reading lay in the interface between their emergent abilities and the tasks they were asked to perform as part of their early instruction.

Readiness as a maturational phenomenon

The concept of readiness grew out of the belief that children's development resulted from intrinsic growth factors that enabled behavior to unfold automatically as the neurophysiological mechanisms matured (Gesell, 1925; see also the review of Hunt, 1964). When it was subsequently discovered in the 1920s, through the widespread use of school surveys, that many first graders were having difficulty learning to read, the assumption that time would prove to be the remedying factor was a natural consequence. Recommendations that reading instruction be delayed became prevalent (Durkin, 1978).

Psychologists and educators became preoccupied with determining *when* children could be expected to profit from instruction in reading. Newly available intelligence quotient tests provided one means of answering that question. Although Durkin documented a number of proposals that established mental-age minimums, the finding of Morphett and Washburne (1931) that beginning instruction when a child had achieved a mental-age score of $6\frac{1}{2}$ years would greatly reduce the incidence of reading failure had the greatest impact. Because the Morphett and Washburne report was questionable in terms of both its scientific rigor and its generalizability, Durkin attributed its impact to both the Zeitgeist and the prominence of Carleton Washburne.

One legacy of the report, bolstered during the 1940s and 1950s by the continued insistence of some influential psychologists (cf. Havinghurst, 1953; Olson, 1949) that reading readiness emerged from maturation, was the widely held belief among both educators and the general public that early instruction could harm children who were not "ready." Kindergartens in some school systems forbade paper and pencils, because the 5-year-olds enrolled were "not ready." Even as late as 1966 Durkin reported that one of the factors which differentiated early readers was having mothers who were not afraid to teach their children to read.

A second, inadvertent legacy was the development of reading readiness tests. The subsequent gradual erosion of faith in intelligence measures, when children of the critical mental age did not always learn to read easily, led researchers to develop instruments designed to measure readiness itself. These measures stimulated the interest in testing, which still dominates educational decision making. Furthermore, the tests defined readiness as achievement on what were to become rather standard tasks of visual discrimination, auditory discrimination, and vocabulary growth. Once defined, these constructs found their way into preschool, kindergarten, and early first-grade curricula. For persons convinced that readiness stemmed from intrinsic growth patterns, there was no requirement that curricular tasks resemble reading. Thus began the fascination with "developmental tasks" (Havinghurst, 1953).

Readiness as the result of early experience

A counter position on readiness, expressed by some members of the educational community, suggested that rather than wait for nature, teachers could nurture readiness in their students. As early as 1925 the National Society for the Study of Education recommended that the preschool, kindergarten, and beginning first-grade years be considered a time to "provide the training and experience which prepare pupils for reading" (cited in Durkin, 1966, p. 6). This recommendation assumes that even though readiness could be nurtured, children

An educational community embracing readiness programs as a panacea for instructional failures resulted in the widespread implementation of sterile and routine educational programs.

through the middle of first grade— mental age of approximately $6^1/_2$—were not ready to read. Therefore, these educators also found the reading readiness tests useful in discriminating groups of children who were "ready" from groups who were not. Unfortunately, large first grades, teachers who had never been trained to teach readiness, and an educational community embracing readiness programs as a panacea for instructional failures resulted in the widespread implementation of sterile and routine educational programs (Durkin, 1978).

Shortly after the appearance of the early readiness tests, Gates and his associates challenged the prevailing concept of readiness. In 1936 research by Gates and Bond indicated that (a) correlations between mental age and reading achievement did not support the interpretation of a critical period for beginning reading, (b) that children's ability to profit from instruction partly depended on the nature of the reading program, and (c) that tutorial interventions could be instituted to enable children failing in reading to achieve success. Three years later, Gates, Bond, and Russell conducted a comprehensive study in which they examined the predictive ability of methods for assessing reading. Readiness tests proved to be of little value.

64 Readiness testing and readiness instruction persisted and continued to persist. Durkin suggested that the prevalence of workbooks, faith in test scores, and the conservative nature of schools are responsible for sustaining the popularity of these practices, even though their effectiveness remains unverified.

Readiness as the interface between children's abilities and task demands

The Russian launching of Sputnik I in October of 1957 inaugurated what promised to be a new era in American education. Educators and psychologists redesigned curricula and reinterpreted many learning concepts, among them the concept of readiness. Although the emphases changed, a revolution in the understanding of readiness was still some years away. But this renewed interest in education among some of America's leading psychologists, educators, and consumers provided the impetus for the significant gains to follow.

Acceptance of interactionism

Perhaps the crucial difference between the emerging position on readiness and those that preceded it was the acceptance of interactionism. Not only did the emphasis in studies of child development begin to focus on the interaction between hereditary and maturational factors and environmental experience (Bruner, 1960; Piaget, 1948, English edition 1973) but learning also came to be viewed as the result of an interaction between the child's abilities and the task's demands (Ausubel, 1959). Attempts to find suitable intervention strategies that might affect the later learning of young preschoolers, especially those who were culturally different and/or deprived, developed into nationwide experimental projects.

Enthusiasm rapidly dampened with the finding that early intervention had failed (Jensen, 1969) or at least had failed to lead to significant, long-term gains. Although national attention had been directed toward improving schooling, educators responded unimaginatively to the challenge and little sustained change resulted. In some instances, readiness instruction was begun earlier or reading instruction was started in kindergarten, but methods and materials used to teach reading remained essentially unaltered.

Revised concept of readiness

Durkin (1968) offered and had some success in gaining popularity for a revised concept of readiness which used the interactionist perspective. Readiness understood as the result of both maturation and experience was necessarily teachable in some measure. Furthermore, emphasis on the *relation* between the child's competence and the task's demand had two consequences. First, instructional decisions had to be individualized. Second, variations in methodology were called for. By teaching the child skills associated with reading the teacher could examine the match between the child and instructional interventions. It was no longer possible to ask the question of whether or not the child was ready. One had to ask, "Ready for what?" Consequently, knowledge of a child's score on a readiness test was not so helpful as watching the child's responses to a varity of educational encounters. The profound change that occurred, and that continues to receive increasing acceptance, was that *"readiness instruction . . . was viewed as reading instruction in its earliest stages"* (Durkin, 1978, p. 169). Reading was viewed as the cumulative acquisition of its component skills, rather than as being discontinuous with readiness.

Several aspects of Durkin's position distinguish it from the orientation which was to follow. First, it accepts the fundamental importance of readiness for successful reading performance in much the same way that parents accept that their children's arms and legs are not long enough to enable them to ride bicycles. Second, the focus remains on the constructs of readiness identified by the early readiness tests—visual discrimination, auditory discrimination, and vocabulary development. Finally, the assumption is made that early reading begins with early instruction. Durkin's (1966) longitudinal studies of children who read early focused on the instructional aspects of reading development rather than on children's learning. For example, Durkin emphasized that preschool reading resulted from help or instruction by parents or older siblings playing school. She concluded that the key element in a child's learning to read before entering school is a supportive, stimulating mother. This emphasis on instruction rather than learning continues to characterize Durkin's later work in redefining readiness.

EVOLUTION OF CHILD READING

The impetus for improved explanations of learning gathered momentum through-out the 1960s and 1970s. Although they have affected educational practice only marginally, substantial strides have been made in the understanding of how children learn. (For an historical overview of learning theory during the last 20 years see Greeno, 1980.) Primary among the changes in the view of learning over the last 2 decades has been the shifting emphasis from models that view learning as the acquisition of bits of information that become integrated into knowledge to assimilative models.

In assimilation or schema theory, learning is seen as an elaboration of past experience. Children actively attribute meaning to objects and experience based on what they already know. They also select, organize, enrich, and retrieve what they experience. This revised understanding of learning has led to a significant departure from traditional models by emphasizing learning rather than teaching. As a result, research on what Gibson (1970) calls the "ontogeny" of reading and what I am referring to as the *evolution* of reading has proliferated.

There appear to be at least two major developments in the evolution of reading ability (Schwartz, 1977). First, children begin to interpret print holistically. Later, they acknowledge its alphabetic nature and gradually begin to show concern— often with instruction—for the internal composition of words. There appears to be a relation between reading proficiency and the ability to subordinate graphic knowledge to meaning—although good readers continue to be aware of and responsive to the surface features of text (Liberman, Liberman, Mattingly, & Shankweiler, 1980).

Child reading as a spontaneous development

For some time it was thought that reading began with formal instruction during the first few years of schooling and was successfully mastered only after children had attained certain prerequisite skills. These prerequisite skills have been defined by various authors as visual and auditory discrimination; sequencing ability; vocabulary knowledge; and even indices of concrete operational reasoning, such as conservation, seriation, and class inclusion (cf. Elkind, 1978). However, more recently it has been recognized that although some reading skills may be related to concrete operational or perceptual behaviors, these behaviors are not prerequisite to beginning reading.

Ironically, Piaget's theory, which has been cited so frequently as evidence that reading ability must await the onset of concrete operational reasoning, provides evidence for an interpretation of early reading as a continuous, spontaneous, and gradual development. According to the tenets of genetic epistemology (Gallagher & Reid, in press; Piaget, 1977), children's ability to interpret symbols begins as early as 18 to 24 months, not with the onset of concrete operations, but as one of two major characteristics of preoperational thinking. Early symbolic behavior is revealed in children's use of deferred imagery, language, play, and drawing.

Early reading originates in the same kind of adaptive behavior that motivates all other kinds of learning and is closely related to the development of oral language.

Furthermore, young children's understanding is symbolic and not simply pictorial (Gibson, 1970).

Early reading originates in the same kind of adaptive behavior that motivates all other kinds of learning and is closely related to the development of oral language (as well as other symbolic abilities). Reinforcement is internal and results from the intrinsic joys of having reduced uncertainty and increased cognitive economy (Gibson, 1970). Children are continually active in their searches for structure and regularity. Furthermore, it seems that it is discovery (rather than directed attention or didactic intervention) which leads to transfer (Bloom & Lahey, 1978; Gibson, 1970; Miller, 1965). As Durkin's (1966) studies indicated, children who learned to read early *asked* their parents and siblings about print. It was children's curiosity and not parental ambition that led to reading among preschoolers.

There appear to be several strands of reading that have their roots in early development and continue to develop and interweave until, apparently, they become consolidated with the achievement of fluent reading. Although children's earliest knowledge of printed symbols seems to derive from struggling to make sense of print in their environments, side benefits also appear to accrue. For example, children gain some familiarity with the alphabetic nature of writing and the conventions associated with text.

Children's earliest reading

Although some children appear to be more interested than others and to profit from greater exposure and stimulation than others, nearly all children learn to recognize some words by sight prior to school entrance and reading instruction. Children's earliest words are usually those which are encountered frequently and which are heavily embedded in situational and contextual cues. Street signs, labels, and store logos tend to be recognized by very young children. In tests of over 1,000 children ages 3 to 7, for example, Reid, Hresko, and Hammill (1981) have yet to find a single child who was not able to recognize the McDonald's sign. Most of the children studied, even those from low-income families, recognized store names, toothpaste packages, and cereal labels.

The earliest reading is somewhat arbitrary and egocentric and in most ways parallels the development of oral language. Children, for example, go through a period of overgeneralization when they read all toothpaste labels as Crest, car dealer logos as Ford, and store signs as K-Mart. Only gradually do they learn to differentiate K-Mart from Woolco and McDonald's from Burger King. Although children are responding to more than the print, Goodman (1980) has shown that children are not fooled by the red, white, and blue of the Pepsi-Cola label. When asked where it says Pepsi, children point to the print. Preschool children also become able to read frequently encountered words that are removed from the context in which they are usually found. Hiebert (1978) demonstrated that words such as *milk* and *cookie* can be read by many preschool children when the words are simply printed on cards.

Response to discourse

Young children also learn to interpret print in connected discourse. Both Goodman (1980) and Reid et al. (1981) have

indicated that 2- 3-, and 4-year-old children are generally competent in orienting a book, newspaper, magazine, or birthday card properly. Many know that the story does not begin on the first page and turn the first two or three pages to reach the place where it says, "Once upon a time . . . ." (Goodman, 1980). Children frequently will recite favorite stories as their parents read to them or supply words and phrases appropriately. Knowledge that one reads from left to right also develops early, as does understanding of the movement from top to bottom. Most children even recognize that it is the writing that is being read aloud. When asked, "Where should I begin reading?", it is not atypical for a 3-year-old child to answer, "Here, with the ABCs." Approximately 75% of the 3- and 4-year-old children studied by Reid et al. (1981) responded to greeting cards (of all varieties) by singing, "Happy Birthday" and read letters and postcards as saying, "Dear John." All of these activities, both in the interpretation of words and discourse, also provide children with the opportunity to learn the vocabulary of print (i.e., *word, letter, page, read*) (Goodman, 1980).

Knowledge of word structure

What exactly children are learning about the structure of words and English orthography during these preschool years is less well documented. Children gradually come to learn the names of the alphabet and numerals, and to write and spell some simple and familiar words (Read, 1975; Reid et al., 1981). Mason (1980) found a developmental sequence which began with children's ability to discriminate letters, followed by their understanding that the letters provided

68

clues used by readers, and finally that sounds of oral language were related to those letters. This development appears to be more closely related to instruction from parents, preschool teachers, older siblings, and even television programs than the forms of child reading previously discussed.

In summary, child reading appears, therefore, to begin when children attain the ability to respond to printed symbols. Young children, in their efforts to make sense of the world, use their knowledge of oral language to make guesses about the meaning of print. They also ask for information about the meaning of print and come to recognize words and groups of words that have particular meaning for them. Most children also become acquainted with some of the conventions of print, such as left-right orientation and opening and closing statements. Many also learn to recognize some letters of the alphabet and some numerals, although how much they learn about the role those elements play in the composition of words is unclear.

Attention to graphic stimuli

Very young children will often open a book and recite what they remember of the familiar story. They are proud of their ability to "read." However, later these same children recognize that the words they are "reading" must have some relation to the words in the text. At this point, many will argue that they can no longer read. Emphasis on the code seems to develop among many children at about age 5 or 6, coincidental with beginning reading instruction.

Although reading errors among begin-

ning first-grade children are consistent with the grammatical and semantic context (Weber, 1970a, 1970b), the number of graphemic errors increases throughout the course of the school year. This shift probably reflects children's natural tendency to construct meaning from print by making use of what they know about oral language and their progressive response to instruction in reading. They become aware that not any word will do: it must be the right word. Among low-ability children, this shift does not occur (Biemiller, 1970), which suggests that it constitutes the development of a more sophisticated strategy. It may be that rather than adding graphemic analysis as an additional aspect of decoding, poor readers increase their attention to orthography at the expense of monitoring meaning (Schwartz, 1977).

Gibson (1970), in an overview of the work she and her students were conducting, noted that 3-year-old children can separate pictures from writing, numerals, and scribbles. By age 4 children could also separate scribbles from writing. Their error patterns suggested that letters were discriminated based on distinctive features which, although shared by different pairs of letters, yield a unique pattern for every individual letter. However, even 6-year-old children had difficulty distinguishing words. The white spaces between words were not understood as constituting boundaries. Children ignored those spaces and chose groups of letters as representing word units. Letter patterns were increasingly well detected with age and schooling, and by third grade, children were able to discriminate permissible from nonpermissible combinations.

Liberman et al. (1980) have hypothesized that knowing how to combine the letters into units appropriate for speech is one aspect of reading skill that separates fluent from beginning readers and develops rapidly at about age 6. Poor readers fail to use phonological representations in their reading, while good readers appear to achieve a higher level of linguistic awareness. Of course, Liberman et. al. believe, as does Gibson (1970; 1976), that reading depends on the child's acquiring spoken language. Later, as the child learns to differentiate graphic symbols, they must be mapped onto speech sounds. The tendency among young children to point to the three words in Kellogg's Raisin Bran while saying *ce-re-al* (Goodman, 1980) may be a primitive beginning of such mapping.

An opposing point of view, perhaps best exemplified by the works of Smith (1975) and Goodman (1976), suggests that reading occurs by relating meaning directly to print, in the same sense that one need not use a verbal intermediary to recognize a chair. These authors, and others of a similar persuasion, argue that children develop linguistic awareness and phonological processing strategies as a consequence of instruction. They suggest that such strategies are not inherent or indeed even helpful in reading. Whether meaning is apprehended directly or whether a translation to a phonological representation is necessary for comprehension is an issue that is not likely to be resolved for some time (Kolers, Wrolstad, & Bouma, 1979); although knowledge of the component relations within words appears to be necessary at some level (Gibson, 1970). What is important is that children begin to recognize the alphabet and its functions during their preschool years. Whether a

shift to graphemic decoding strategies is instructionally induced or spontaneously generated, it has probably been evolving for some time.

SUMMARY AND CONCLUSIONS

The changing nature of readiness

The concept of readiness gained recognition at the turn of the century and was soon used to explain reading failure. At first readiness was viewed as the outgrowth of automatic, neurophysiological development. Although a group of educators were quick to respond that readiness could be fostered in children, they were apparently convinced that it could be fostered only after children were "ready." A synthesizing position on readiness which viewed it as the interface between children's abilities and task demands was popularized by Durkin in the 1960s. Although this interactionist position signaled some important advances (e.g., that it was more profitable to present reading tasks to children and observe their ability to learn them than to give global tests of readiness), it still (a) focused on instruction rather than learning, (b) instructed children in predominantly perceptual rather than linguistic tasks, and (c) assumed that a period of readiness is required before reading instruction can be profitable.

The revolution in thinking about the concept of readiness did not occur with Sputnik, as promised, but developed with the rise of psycholinguistics. With Chomsky's (1965) description of language development came a recognition that children were not cognitively biding their time during the preschool years develop-

70 ing the muscular and ocular coordination that would enable them to benefit from instruction at age 5 or 6. Instead children were actively seeking to make sense of their physical world and their social environments, especially the linguistic environment. They were selecting, guessing, testing, and generating categories and systems of words and knowledge. What was striking about that realization was that no one was teaching them. Children were acquiring oral language spontaneously and were applying that knowledge to the interpretation of print as well.

Evolution as a more appropriate concept

The need for a concept of readiness evaporated. Children did not develop a series of skills whose later metamorphosis enabled them to read. They began learning to read (learning about the vocabulary and strategies and processes of reading) through trial and error, through selecting, guessing, testing, and generating categories and systems of words and knowledge—just as they were organizing their oral language experiences.

Child reading was then interpreted as a gradual, spontaneous evolution beginning with the holistic attribution of meaning to print and later, apparently with instruction, becoming refined in such a way as to enable the reader to become knowledgeable about the component elements of words (and perhaps their relation to oral language). Apparent in spontaneous attempts at reading is that children apply their knowledge of syntax and semantics to their interpretation of print. Only later do children focus seriously on the graphemic cues. Reading occurs through the progressive refinement of successive approximations. There is no readiness different from reading itself and reading is primarily cognitive and linguistic and not visual and perceptual.

A significant disadvantage of the concept of readiness, which continues to exist in all its forms in today's schools, is that it interferes with the development of children's reading ability. As Durkin (1978) noted, most schools that have readiness programs have them for all children. What tends to vary is the amount of time that children wait until instruction in reading is begun. Readiness tests, which are still popular, are used as measures to determine in a global way who is ready (for what is ignored) and who is not. Additionally, programs that begin with readiness activities are discontinuous with children's spontaneous development. These programs fail to capitalize on the knowledge (of both printed and oral language) that children bring with them to school.

Advantages of viewing development as constituting a continuous evolution of reading behaviors include parsimony and instructional implications. In regard to parsimony, characteristics of child reading ability appear to be consistent with children's early cognitive development (Ausubel, 1959; Bruner, 1960; Piaget, 1977) and with their development of other language abilities. Halliday (1975), for example, noted in his study of Nigel's language acquisition that there was an early period of arbitrary, egocentric language development, followed by successive approximations of the phonology and lexicon of his mother tongue. The same kind of development is apparent in written language. Read (1975), for example, described children's early writing as primarily personal and evolving gradually to conform with the adult standard, again through successive approximations. Reading, therefore, does not appear to require a special cognitive system, but rather is interrelated with and develops according to the same constraints as other cognitive and linguistic abilities. Consequently there is no more need to separate child reading from later reading development than there is to separate child (oral) language from later linguistic development. One is simply a more primitive form which gradually evolves into the other.

Finally, the educational implications of viewing child reading as the beginning of a continuous evolution are (a) the interrelatedness of cognitive and linguistic functions and (b) the need for continuity between the child's knowledge and the program he or she is offered in school. These implications suggest that programs in which all aspects of language functioning are stimulated simultaneously may prove useful. Although attention to the surface features of both oral and written language appears to be needed, initial instruction must include some experiences with reading that enable children to sustain or develop a schema for reading that recognizes that the purpose of print is to convey meaning. Instruction which is continuous with the earlier, spontaneous developments of child reading provides an alternative to repetitious drills that currently characterize initial instruction for children who experience problems in learning to read.

REFERENCES

Ausubel, D.P. Viewpoints from related disciplines: Human growth and development. *Teachers College Record*, 1959, *60*, 245–254.

Biemiller, A. The development of the use of graphic and contextual information as children learn to read. *Reading Research Quarterly*, 1970, *6*, 75–96.

Bloom, L., & Lahey, M. *Language development and language disorders*. New York: John Wiley and Sons, 1978.

Bruner, J. *The process of education*. Cambridge, Mass.: Harvard University Press, 1960.

Chomsky, N. Aspects of the theory of syntax. Cambridge, Mass.: M.I.T. Press, 1965.

Durkin, D. *Children who read early: Two longitudinal studies*. New York: Columbia University Teachers College Press, 1966.

Durkin, D. When should children begin to read? In, *Innovation and change in reading instruction: Sixty-seventh yearbook of the National Society for the Study of Education*. Chicago: University of Chicago Press, 1968.

Durkin, D. *Teaching them to read*. Boston: Allyn & Bacon, 1978.

Elkind, D. Stages in the development of reading. Paper presented at the 8th annual symposium of the Jean Piaget Society, Philadelphia, May 1978.

Gallagher, J.M., & Reid, D.K. *The learning theory of Piaget and Inhelder*. Monterey, Calif.: Brooks/Cole Publishing Company, in press.

Gates, A.I., & Bond, G. Reading readiness: A study of factors determining success and failure in beginning reading. *Teachers College Record*, 1936, *37*, 679–685.

Gates, A.I., Bond, G.I., & Russell, D.H. *Methods of determining reading readiness*. New York: Bureau of Publications, Columbia University Teachers College Press, 1939.

Gesell, A.L. *The mental growth of the preschool child*. New York: Macmillan, 1925.

Gibson, E.J. The ontogeny of reading. *American Psychologist*, 1970, *25*, 136–143.

Gibson, E.J. Learning to read. In H. Singer & R. Ruddell (Eds.), *Theoretical models and processes of reading*. Newark, Del.: International Reading Association, 1976.

Goodman, K. Reading: A psycholinguistic guessing game. In H. Singer & R. Ruddell (Eds.), *Theoretical models*

72

and processes of reading. Newark, Del.: International Reading Association, 1976.

Goodman, Y. Roots of literacy. In M. Douglas (Ed.), *44th Yearbook of the Claremont Reading Conference.* Claremont, Calif.: Claremont Reading Conference, 1980.

Greeno, J.G. Psychology of learning, 1960–1980: One participant's observations. *American Psychologist,* 1980, *35,* 713–728.

Halliday, M.A.K. Learning how to mean. In E.H. Lenneberg & E. Lenneberg (Eds.), *Foundations of language development: A multidisciplinary approach.* New York: Academic Press, 1975.

Havinghurst, R. *Human development and education.* New York: Longmans, Green, and Co. 1953.

Hiebert, E.H. Preschool children's understanding of written language. *Child Development,* 1978, *49,* 1231–1234.

Hunt, J.M. The psychological basis for using preschool enrichment as an antidote for cultural deprivation. *Merrill-Palmer Quarterly,* 1964, *10,* 209–248.

Jensen, A. How much can we boost IQ and scholastic achievement? *Harvard Educational Review,* 1969, *4,* 37–47.

Kolers, P.A., Wrolstad, M.E., & Bouma, H. *Processing visible language.* Vol. 1. New York: Plenum Press, 1979.

Liberman, I.Y., Liberman, A.M., Mattingly, I.G., & Shankweiler, D. Orthography and the beginning reader. In J. Kavanagh & R. Venezky (Eds.), *Orthography, reading, and dyslexia.* Baltimore: University Park Press, 1980.

Mason, J. When do children begin to read: An exploration of four year old children's letter and word reading competencies. *Reading Research Quarterly,* 1980, *15,* 203–227.

Miller, G.A. Some preliminaries to psycholinguistics. *American Psychologist,* 1965, *20,* 15–20.

Morphett, M.V., & Washburne, C. When should children begin to read? *Elementary School Journal,* 1931, *31,* 496–503.

Olson, W. *Child development.* Boston: D. C. Heath and Co., 1949.

Piaget, J. *To understand is to invent.* New York: Viking Press, 1973 (French edition, 1948).

Piaget, J. *The development of thought: Equilibration of cognitive structure.* New York: Viking Press, 1977 (French edition, 1975).

Read, C. Lessons to be learned from the preschool orthographer. In E.H. Lenneberg & E. Lenneberg (Eds.), *Foundations of language development: A multidisciplinary approach.* New York: Academic Press, 1975.

Reid, D.K., Hresko, W.P., & Hammill, D.D. *Test of early reading.* Austin, Tex.: Pro-Ed, 1981.

Schwartz, R.M. Strategic processes in beginning reading. *Journal of Reading Behavior,* 1977, *9,* 17–26.

Smith, F. *Comprehension and learning: A conceptual framework for teachers.* New York: Holt, Rinehart and Winston, 1975.

Weber, R. First-graders use of grammatical context in reading. In H. Levin & J. Williams (Eds.), *Basic studies in reading.* New York: Basic Books, 1970 (a).

Weber, R. A linguistic analysis of first-grade reading errors. *Reading Research Quarterly,* 1970, *5,* 427–451. (b)

Developmental Issues in Written Language

Bonnie E. Litowitz, Ph.D.
Associate Professor
Department of Communicative
Disorders, and
Department of Linguistics
Northwestern University
Evanston, Illinois

WRITING IS a late-acquired activity that follows speech phylogenetically, developmentally, and structurally. Writing appears comparatively late in the cultural history of mankind (and not in all cultures); it follows considerable cognitive and linguistic development in the psychological history of each individual; and it is built on preexisting structures of cognition and language, recoding and extending them beyond their previous limits.

The priority of the spoken over the written medium (Lyons, 1968) by linguists, anthropologists, teachers, and therapists has resulted in more knowledge about oral language than written language. The nature of writing must be explored more fully to help young writers (those of any age who are beginning to write). This article suggests that writing disorders can only be understood against a background of knowledge about writing as a complex activity. Furthermore, this knowledge is best gained by a careful analysis of both the writer and what he or

0271-8294/81/0012-0073$2.00

73

74 she brings to the task, as well as the nature of writing and the task itself.

Writing is a complex activity in at least two ways. First, writing is complex because it subsumes previous skills and processes. Identification of the underlying processes and their contribution to the activity of writing adds not only to knowledge of writing but also to the ability to assess latent problems. These problems, although not particular to writing, may nonetheless manifest themselves in writing. Writing is also complex because it requires an indirect, abstract way of relating between the writer and his or her world. The alphabetic-phonetic writing system does not directly record experience. It recodes previously coded experience at a distance from another person (the reader) in a new and highly elaborated logical and structural form (the text). This second notion of complexity is based on writing as a new type of representational system. Those writers whose basic underlying processes or integrities are sufficient to engage in writing but who cannot deal with the added demands caused by the complexity of writing can be assessed.

There are two major groups of problems concerning writing disorders: (a) due to deficits in underlying processes required for writing, and (b) due to the additional complexities inherent in written representation. Disorders of both kinds have been discussed elsewhere (Johnson & Myklebust, 1967; Myklebust, 1965, 1973). The first type will only be reviewed here while major emphasis will be on exploring the nature of writing to more fully understand the second type.

A third group of problems includes disabilities due to instructional deficits. Students require instruction to master writing, either through direct intervention or opportunities to discover. Students who have not had appropriate instruction may produce written products judged to be below their teachers' expectations. Students who enter basic writing classes in some colleges and universities may not have underlying disorders or specific writing disabilities but rather instructional deficits. Remedial course work could be directed at providing basic instruction (Shaughnessy, 1977). During the process of evaluation it is important to take a student's history of the amount and kind of instruction previously received. However, it may still be difficult to differentially diagnose the three types of problems outlined here. Perhaps the only way to isolate these specific disorders from instructional deficits is in diagnostic teaching where a teacher can observe the student's responses to differential interventions.

LANGUAGE HIERARCHY

The ability to write follows developmentally and structurally the abilities to listen, speak, and read. Johnson and Myklebust (1967) and Myklebust (1965, 1973) have posited a hierarchy of language abilities to illustrate this point (Figure 1).

The development of abilities in the language hierarchy relies on the initially intact receptive language capacity. If there is any problem with the language that the child acquires receptively (e.g., due to sensory impairment, auditory memory deficits, or auditory discrimina-

Written Expression
Reading (Receptive)

Oral Expression
Oral Receptive

Fig. 1. The language hierarchy.

tion problems), then all capacities above this level will be affected. This first level in the hierarchy will be needed for the next level, oral expression, which combines receptive language information with motor expression. Problems at this level (e.g., articulation difficulties or sequencing problems that disturb syntactic patterning) may affect higher levels of the language hierarchy.

Abilities

Myriad cognitive or psychological abilities are subsumed under the need for basic oral language capacities, both receptive and expressive. The ability to perceive and therefore discriminate auditory stimuli and to classify and categorize these into significant groups is necessary to learn the distinctive, meaningful sounds of a particular language. Similarly, the ability to combine these sound patterns into meaningfully sequenced groups is necessary to form words and sentences.

Less obvious perhaps are the requirements for other (i.e., nonauditory) perceptions, selective attention, and categorization, which imply the ability to solve problems, learn strategies and rules, and apply them. These other abilities are necessary to understand the world of experience that language codes. An example of the latter might be a child who has difficulty in the visual-perceptual discrimination of lemons and oranges. He or

she will not be able to classify these as subclasses of a larger class, fruits (Anglin, 1977; Brown, 1978). Even if the child has the ability to learn the linguistic code, it will be meaningless unless connected correctly to perceived, conceptualized, and remembered experiences.

Problems observed in one area may actually be more fundamental. For example, a generalized perceptual or sequencing deficit or a specifically linguistic perceptual or sequencing deficit (i.e., auditory discrimination and sequencing for language units) may be found. Difficulties in segmenting and sequencing language may also reflect difficulties in a nonverbal performance (e.g., in understanding causes and effects, series, or steps in a plan).

Therefore it is necessary to examine all aspects of the oral language systems that might affect writing performance. In addition, problems the writer may have in nonlinguistic experience must be explored, with the realization that the verbal system codes a nonverbal reality (Johnson & Myklebust, 1967).

When children move up the language hierarchy from oral to nonoral media, they move further from nonverbal reality. A bar has been added to Figure 1 to mark this change. Whereas oral language codes reality in a system of arbitrary, conventional, auditorily perceived verbal signs, written language codes, not the underlying reality, but the previous system of arbitrary signs by means of a new system. This new system is equally arbitrary and conventional, but it is visual. Like those abilities below the bar, these *re*coding capacities have receptive and expressive aspects. Reading involves the receptive

75

76 ability to deal with the second-order sign system.

Coding

Therefore the four levels of the language hierarchy comprise two sets: the first, verbally coding experience; the second, recoding the first. Within each set are two levels, the first a *de*coding capacity, the second, an *en*coding capacity. Coding abilities in relation to recoding abilities, and decoding abilities, in relation to encoding abilities, are developmentally prior because they are easier and require less work in processing time. Therefore they are faster and can cover more material in less time. Thus listening and reading are easier ways to obtain information

---

Listening and reading are easier ways to obtain information than speaking and writing.

---

than speaking and writing. People can hear more and faster than they can speak, and read more and faster than they can write; it takes more effort (work) to speak than listen, write than read. From this perspective it is possible to generalize about other encoding and recoding abilities. For example, finger spelling in the sign language of the deaf, Morse Code, and seamen's flag signals should be even more demanding because these represent encoding tasks at still a third level of recoding. These examples demonstrate another way decoding and coding occur prior to encoding and recoding at different levels, namely, structurally. The

term *structurally prior* means that later abilities are built on the structural units of the previous level.

REPRESENTATION

The structure of the linguistic sign (word) was clearly stated by de Saussure (1959), not as the relationship between a word and a thing, but as the relationship between an acoustic sound-image and a concept. Many cognitive and psychological abilities enter into the relationship between concepts and things (e.g., selective attention, perception, categorization, memory, and problem solving). Language certainly has a major, although often-disputed, role (Bruner, 1973; Piaget, 1955; Vygotsky, 1962, 1978). Nevertheless, in writing, the written visual signs represent the acoustic image and only through its mediation, the concept.

This "second-order" (Vygotsky, 1978) or "second-degree" of symbolization (Vygotsky, 1962) is a peculiarity of an alphabetic writing system. Of the major types of writing systems, pictographs are at one end of the spectrum. They represent reality directly. Pictographs and acoustic-images can be considered as alternate representations of reality. Ideographic writing, where a grapheme (i.e., a unit in the visual writing system) represents an idea or word, is midway between representing reality directly and representing language. However, syllabic and phonetic writing no longer represent reality or concepts directly but instead represent the sound-image itself. Syllabaries divide the sound-image into larger units than phonetic systems (Chao, 1970; Gelb, 1963). It is possible to analyze acoustic sound images further than alphabetic writing; Initial Teaching Alphabets are an attempt in this direction (Downing, 1965).

The implications of different types of writing systems were not lost on Rousseau as early as 1761:

The first way of writing is not to paint the sounds, but the objects themselves, either directly, as the Mexicans did, or by allegorical figures, as the Egyptians used to do. This state corresponds to the 'passionate' language. . . . The second way is to represent words and propositions by conventional characters, which can only occur . . . amongst an entire people united by common laws. . . . Such is the writing of the Chinese, which is in essence a way of painting sounds and of speaking to the eyes. The third way is to decompose the speaking voice into a certain number of elementary parts, either vocal or articulated, with which one can form all imaginable words and syllables. This way of writing . . . must have been imagined by a commercial people (who needed a set of) characters common to all languages. To do this is not exactly to paint speech, it is to analyze it. (p. 507)

Thus to be able to write requires an additional kind of analysis of speech than that required for speaking.

Visual-graphemic system

Writing requires analysis of those units in the acoustic stream that correspond to already established units in the visual-graphemic system. Analysis and establishment of units in the graphemic system require abilities in visual discrimination, memory, and categorization. In addition, writing requires a motoric act, which includes the design of characters or letters and spacing between letters and significant groups of letters, as well as abilities in

spatial direction and sequencing. The temporal (auditory) linearity of speech must be resymbolized into the spatial (visual) linearity of written language.

The visual-spatial-symbol system captures more from the auditory system than the letter-to-sound correspondences. There are graphic symbols for nonletter phenomena such as spaces and punctuation for intonation, pitch, stress, and junctures in speech. Furthermore, the correspondence between the visual-graphemic and auditory-phonemic systems is initially arbitrary. Distinctive features in the visual system do not correspond to significant features in the phonemic system (Gibson & Levin, 1975). For example, /k/ and /g/ are phonically close but visually distinct, although /p/ and /b/ are close in both systems. Nonetheless, there is no visual feature (e.g., straight line, open curve) that corresponds to a particular auditory feature (e.g., voicing, bilabial articulation, stridence); neither is there a temporal feature (e.g, length of juncture) with a spatial feature (e.g., size of space). Nor in English is there a one-to-one correspondence between a grapheme (once learned) and a sound class (Chao, 1970). The difficulty that children have with spelling bears witness to the distance between the graphemic and phonemic systems. In addition, analytic writing systems require that multiple sequencing and combinatory patterns be learned, which is another cause for spelling errors.

Many authors (Beers & Henderson, 1977; Read, 1971, 1975) suggest that children actively hypothesize a series of rules of graphemic-phonemic correspondence, successively coming closer and closer to the adult rules. This is accomplished in

78

much the same way as researchers have suggested that children master oral language in general, such as phonology, morphology, syntax (de Villiers & de Villiers, 1978), or cognitive logical structures (Piaget & Inhelder, 1969). This approach envisions learning to spell as a problem-solving task, part of the larger tasks of reading and writing. Early attempts to spell (or write) should not be seen as failed or partial adult solutions but as complete and internally consistent early solutions (preoperational logical thought or early grammar).

As in speaking, in spelling and writing the child hypothesizes strategies or rules based on given information. However, instruction plays a key role in these later activities. Different curricula in spelling and in reading will influence spelling by suggesting preferred strategies. For example, the teaching of the alphabet enters into early strategies of children's spelling as they use the name of the letter to represent the sound. Later, visual information will also become incorporated, for example, /f/ can be represented by *f* or *ph* (Beers & Henderson, 1977).

The following curriculum sequence is often used and can be seen to affect strategies: the teacher explains the alphabet or visual-graphemic systems; those sounds that correspond directly (e.g., *fan, dan, pan*); the rules to cover those that do not but are rule-governed; and finally "sight words" that defy correspondence or other rules. To learn sight words individuals must disregard the analysis of sound-images and correspondences to graphemic-images and instead learn the graphemic-image as if it were a "pictograph" or "ideograph" of the whole word.

To extend the sight-word approach to all words would bypass the difficulties of analysis and correspondence rules but burden visual memory (as do all pictographic writing systems). Alphabetic systems trade off a small inventory of graphemic units, which are easy to remember, with complex rules of combinations, which are difficult to learn.

Visual-manual representational system

Besides visual-auditory and spatial-temporal correspondences, writing is a visual-manual representational system. Disorders of manual, expressive output in writing are not discussed here (see Johnson & Myklebust, 1967; Luria, 1959; Myklebust, 1965; Weigl, 1975). Therefore writing shares a common source with drawing; both begin from the need to *re*-present that something else by leaving a trace on paper that stands for something else (see Gardner's notion of "rendering," 1980). The resulting scribbles are the earliest stages of both drawing (Kellogg & O'Dell, 1967) and writing (Hildreth, 1936; Luria, 1978; Vygotsky, 1978). Writing systems, whether pictographic or alphabetic, demand that a conventional visual sign system be learned for representation. The postscribbling divergence between the development of drawing and the development of writing indicates that children are aware of the difference in these two representational activities. They recognize that the goal of the former is to represent reality, that of the latter, to represent speech.

Semiotic system

Although Piaget called attention to the common source and similarities in all representational activities (e.g., oral language, play, drawing), Vygotsky (1962, 1978) illuminated the nature of the extension of the semiotic function with the acquisition of second-order symbolic systems such as writing (and also math).

In analyzing representation by levels or degrees of the semiotic system, the differences between writing and speaking are clear. More generally, both writing and speaking represent ideas. There is no point in learning either first- or second-order linguistic systems, unless it is to "forget" it (i.e., make it automatic and unconscious), so that ideas can be transmitted.

Both speaking and writing undergo the same spiral of development. First, conscious attention is used to acquire the linguistic system. It then becomes unconsciously and automatically used in the pursuit of another consciously attended problem, for example, to remember someone's name. A final stage is the reemergence of conscious attention to language and its uses, an aspect of metalinguistic awareness. Vygotsky claimed that one benefit of writing was to help focus awareness on grammar, words, and logic, thereby influencing reading, speaking, and thinking (1962). Specifically concerning writing, Vygotsky stated that in early writing "written signs are entirely first-order symbols . . . , directly denoting objects or actions, and the child has yet to reach second-order symbolism" (1978, p. 115). However, after acquiring second-order symbolism the writer acts as if second-order symbols were first-order symbols, directly transforming ideas into writing.

One of the major difficulties of early

With increasing awareness of the limitations of their writing abilities . . . children become less willing to write, much as they lose interest in drawing.

writing is that young writers must focus their conscious attention on the ideas they wish to express while still consciously aware of their less-than-automatic writing skills. Very young children will blissfully forge ahead, unaware of the problem a reader will have because of poor spelling or letter formation. These early pieces of writing will often combine drawing, letters, words, and misspellings but are produced as a true representation of the writer's ideas. With increasing awareness of the limitations of their writing abilities, often accentuated by teachers' comments, children become less willing to write, much as they lose interest in drawing (Gardner, 1980). However, the demands from the children's environment differ. Drawing becomes an optional activity while writing is increasingly required.

The ability to express ideas by means of writing has been called *authoring (authorship)* by Moffett and is distinguished by him from lesser writing skills: drawing and handwriting; transcribing and copying; paraphrasing, summarizing, and plagiarizing; and crafting conventional or given subject matter. These activities are "increasingly difficult for both writer and the teacher of writing" (1979, p. 278). By *authoring* Moffett means "authentic expression of an individual's own ideas—some focused and edited version of inner speech" (1979, p. 278).

80   INNER SPEECH, ORAL LANGUAGE, AND WRITING

The relationship between inner and written speech has been best explained by Vygotsky (1962) and illustrates the connection and also the crucial differences between oral and written language. In an effort to explain the approximately 6-year delay for most children between speaking and writing, Vygotsky offered the following conclusion: writing is abstract compared to the immediacy of spoken language. While written language is like oral language in thought and imagery, its structure and mode of functioning differ.

Differences between oral and written language

In writing children must disengage themselves from the expressive and musical words and intonational qualities of oral speech. They must replace these by images of words (reauditorized and revisualized) that they must consciously (at least at first) call up from memory. In addition, writing is not a social activity, unlike speech, with social interaction, exchange, participation, and feedback. Instead writing is a lonely, isolated act— language addressed to an absent other. Following is Lopate's (1977) description of the differences between oral and written language:

Speech is sociable. Speech has the tendency to rekindle euphoric faith in a social order: with every exchange it knits and reknits the relationship between people. Speech is improvisational, relatively unpremeditated, impulsive; you can open your mouth not knowing exactly what is going to come out or when you are going to stop, but you trust to your adrenalin. The whole body speaks through speech, not only the tongue. Speech rushes on its adrenalized path, it doesn't look back. It is an underselected tape of messages that almost erases itself in its headlong flight. Speech longs to go on forever, for an infinity. The last thing it wants to do is stand still. (p. 24)

In contrast to speaking, writing is a premeditated, intentional, and willed act. It is the product of conscious selection. For the reasons mentioned previously, Lopate concluded that "people are right to be intimidated by writing. Writing is intimidating and kids know it" (1977, p. 24).

Vygotsky (1962) claimed that it is precisely the missing other, this addressing of language to an absent or imaginary or nonexistent person, that is odd for a child. Children cannot see the usefulness of such "disembodied speech," removed from real-life situations and persons. All their actions and interactions with others are embedded in real-life contexts, meeting real-life needs and demands. Oral speech is part of these contexts involving other people; writing is not.

Inner speech

For all the differences between oral and written language, both have a common source in early social dialogue. Early social dialogue becomes separated into social speech for others and inner or private speech for oneself (Figure 2a). Inner speech comes from the same source as social speech but has become internalized. Written language relies on inner speech for its thought and content while still directed to another (an absent other) as is social speech (Figure 2b).

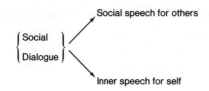

Fig. 2a. The development of oral and inner speech from dialogue.

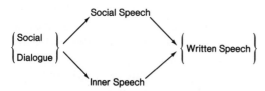

Fig. 2b. The development of written speech.

However, when speech is internalized in inner language, changes take place in its structure. It becomes sense-saturated; subjects drop out; meanings are highly personal. Speech for oneself does not need to state a topic, use socially shared meanings, or even careful logical organization. Written speech, in contrast, is the opposite. While inner speech is structurally condensed, written language must be the most explicit and elaborated, more so than oral speech, which can rely on situational context and participant feedback (Vygotsky, 1962). Figure 3 shows the structural relationships among different types of speech.

Moffett's concept of writing as authoring ("a focused and edited version of inner speech") underscores the source of written language in inner speech. He

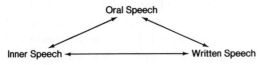

Fig. 3. The relationship of different kinds of speech.

assailed the "superficial view that spelling and punctuating are basic skills, instead of thinking and speaking, and ... the analytic isolation of language units as curriculum units (the phoneme, the word, the sentence, the paragraph)" (1979, p. 278). He stressed that children do not learn writing by bits and pieces as curricula would suggest, but "from the outset, [even] lettering needs to be connected to meaning, to the symbolizing of inner speech" (1979, p. 278).

Even though from the beginning writing is a total activity, the forcing of minimal inner language through highly formal and explicit written forms, imperfectly acquired, is difficult for most early writers. Rosen and Rosen commented on this problem: "Developed writing cannot occur until inner speech is fully developed and by the same token early writing must be aided by external speech" (1973, p. 269). Still they agreed with Vygotsky (1962) and Luria (1978) that once mastered writing can enhance inner language and thought by "transforming [children's] ways of thinking and feeling" (1973, p. 268). Rosen and Rosen stated that "the development of a new medium of expression with its own unique possibilities for enabling children to understand and act in their world" (1973, p. 149) allows the young writer to sift, select and evaluate life. Rosen and Rosen continued: "The result of slow growth over the years [is] the capacity to internalize the world including ourselves and others" (1973, p. 152).

During the course of language development (Figure 2a), all of the functions that speech can serve for the child in a dialogue with an adult become self-func-

81

82 tions. Zaporozhets and Elkonin (1971), Soviet researchers, suggest that all *intra*-psychic functions are *inter*-psychic in origin. For example, using language with an adult to express and refer, to plan, direct, or regulate activities, becomes for the child self-expression, self-reference, self-direction, and self-regulation. The Soviet theorists suggest that just as oral language is learned with another person in a functional context, so too must writing be acquired in a context in which it has a meaningful function. Others have also stressed the functions that writing can serve for the writer. Britton, Burgess, Martin, McLeod, and Rosen (1975) posit three major functional categories (from Jakobson, 1960) for the writing of school-age children (ages 11 to 18): transactional, expressive, and poetic (also see Britton, 1975). For these authors children's developing sense of audience is a major factor in their writing for various functions.

TEXTUALIZATION AND THE ABSENT OTHER

The problem of audience arises out of the difference between speaking and writing in the presence or absence of another. In social dialogue there is, of course, always another; in internalized speech, one treats oneself like another. Writing requires deliberate analytic action (the tying of sounds and images of words to ideas) while at the same time holding the topic and information in mind, all as it needs to be expressed to someone who is not present. Because the absent other may not have all the shared information, which in oral language is present in shared context, written lan-guage must be fully elaborated to provide all the information an absent other might need. The writer must be a "predictor of reactions and act on his predictions" concerning the absent reader (Rosen & Rosen, 1973, p. 265).

Written speech must explain the situation fully to be intelligible to the potential reader; all context must be textualized. According to Vygotsky, textualization requires "deliberate semantics," that is, "deliberate structuring of the web of meaning." Following is Vygotsky's description of textualization:

Communication in writing relies on formal meanings—requires a much greater number of words than oral speech to convey the same idea because it is addressed to an absent person who rarely has the same subject in mind . . . it must be fully deployed . . . syntactic differentiation is at the maximum and expressions are used that would seem unnatural in conversation (1962, p. 100).

Most developmentalists agree that a major developmental movement for the child in acquiring oral language is from situational speech (which is tied to acts, gestures, mimicry, and immediate shared contexts) to decontextualized speech, freed from a specific context in reality (Zaporozhets & Elkonin, 1971, p. 113). Bruner described this progression as the child's "movement toward context-free elaboration" (1975, p. 70). The subsequent and progressive textualization of written language is one of the major distinguishing characteristics differentiating it from oral language (along with the nature of second-order symbolization and the absent other). Learning to create the text demands that the child change from maximally compact and personal inner

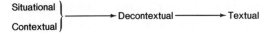

Fig. 4. Direction of language development.

speech to maximally formal and elaborated public speech. The child must learn to progress along the continuum in Figure 4, progressively loading more material into the text so that it can stand independently of the writer or the situation.

Most measures of written language, focusing on the product of writing as opposed to the process or activity of writing, are concerned with textualization. Such measures include number of words per sentence, number of words per clause, number of clauses per terminal-unit (T-unit—one main clause plus whatever subordinate clauses are attached to it), number of T-units per sentence (Hunt, 1975); as well as total number of different words or type-token word ratios, ratio of function words to total words, abstract nouns to total nouns (Geest, Gerstel, Appel, & Tervoort, 1973); and other indices of syntactic maturity (O'Donnell, 1976) or difficulty (Harris, 1977). These authors suggest that as children get older their writing gets longer and more complex, outstripping oral language complexity by fifth grade (O'Donnell, Griffin, & Norris, 1967) or eighth grade (Loban, 1964). The preceding measures are attempts to characterize these facts. Standardized written language tests (e.g., Picture Story Language Test, Myklebust, 1965; Test of Written Language, Hammill & Larsen, 1978) also have attempted to evaluate the semantic changes necessitated by writing (Vygotsky's "deliberate semantics" and "formal meanings").

In writing, syntax becomes more elaborate because of complex clausal constructions involving embeddings, gerunds, relative clauses, adverbial constructions, and complex subordination and coordination. Halliday and Hasan refer to these and to general issues of anaphora (i.e., reference) as cohesive devices that are "relations of meaning that exist within the text, and that define it as a text" (1976, p. 4). These include both vocabulary and grammatical aspects of language. Markers of reference, sometimes called deixis (Fillmore, 1975), note relationships within a particular communicational act.

Developmentally, deictic markers of person (*I, you, he, she, it*), place (*here, there*) and time (*now, then*), demonstratives (*this, that*), and locatives (*up, down, right, left*) are first used situationally, then symbolically (i.e., contextually) and then anaphorically (i.e., textually), following the progression in Figure 4. For example: "Put it *there*" depends on knowledge of the situation and gestures; "Is John *there*?" asked of a person on the telephone can be interpreted purely linguistically; but "I parked my car in the lot and left my keys *there*" refers within the text (Fillmore, 1975, p. 41).

Other authors make similar distinctions: Halliday and Hasan distinguish between exophoric (situational) and endophoric (textual) references and conjunctions that function externally (situationally) or internally (textually) to combine statements. Dever speaks of environmentally versus linguistically conditioned ellipsis (i.e., omission of shared or state material) (1978, p. 187).

A difficulty for young writers is that the same linguistic mechanisms are used in all

84

three "contexts": the pragmatic real world situation; context-free language use; and textual cohesion. Consequently, errors in cohesive ties are frequent and remain, even for older writers. These errors reflect problems with the linguistic devices themselves, the writer's sense of audience, and the added cognitive demands of textual structures.

Both Bruner & Olson (1978) and Olson (1977) stressed the increased cognitive demands and the cognitive benefits of learning to construct texts. Olson (1977) made the following statement:

The bias of written language toward providing definitions, making all assumptions and premises explicit, and observing the formal rules of logic produces an instrument of considerable power for building an abstract and coherent theory of reality. (p. 278)

To master this new instrument requires a change in children's thinking.

Piaget's (1951) analyses of children's constructions of reality indicate the change in logical connectives, reflecting underlying cognitive structural changes. Early reasoning favors juxtaposition and syncretism (i.e., the simple stringing together or overinvolvement of elements in personal, subjective schemas). Early writing reflects this cognitive level by its excessive use of "and," "and so," and run-on sentences. More mature organization depends on "because," "therefore," "however," "previously," "next," and similar words that are only meaningfully available to children of more advanced cognitive stages. In the same way the ability to deal in possibilities, which is a hallmark of formal operational intelligence, is reflected in the full use of modal verbs, tense, and aspect in verb phrases, and other aspects of the linguistic system.

The way propositions are organized and connected requires that the writer bring some concept of text to the activity of writing. Recently text structure has been studied extensively by researchers in reading comprehension and recall. Text-organization, as defined by these authors, may be a useful addition to syntactic measures in evaluating writing and cognition (Mandler & Johnson, 1977; Meyer, 1975; Stein & Nezworski, 1978; Thorndyke, 1977). For example, children have a concept of story (Applebee, 1978) as well as other genres, which they bring to the task of writing. Whether acquired from their reading or other writing experience, a concept of text greatly aids organization and memory.

THE COMPOSING PROCESS

Besides the maximum elaboration of the text, the problem of the absent other or potential reader is a difficulty for representing inner speech in written language. A full understanding of the activity of writing, called the composing process, involves not only the subject matter and the text but also a sense of audience. Gundlach, Litowitz, and Moses (1979) have characterized these as aspects of the composing process (Figure 5).

Some authors (such as Britton et al., 1975) focus on the function of writing for

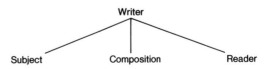

Fig. 5. Three aspects of the composing process.

different audiences (e.g., self, teacher, and friend). They claim that early writing is expressive but becomes transactional as the writer considers another person or poetic when concentrated on the text itself rather than on a reader (Britton, 1975). Other authors suggest that children master different genres or types of texts at different stages of development. These types begin with "interior dialogue" (like egocentric speech) followed by "vocal dialogue" (like socialized speech) through "correspondence," "personal journal," "autobiography," "memoir," "biography," "chronicle," "history," and finally, "science" and "metaphysics" (Moffett, 1968). Such a progression illustrates writing for oneself, then for another who is increasingly abstract and distant.

Topic

Such a linear developmental sequence relies on the acceptance of the notion that children are initially egocentric and only later concerned with communication (Piaget, 1955). However, examples taken from children's early writing do not support this assumption. Instead, observations from writing support the growing body of research that finds that children are not necessarily egocentric—although they often are (Ervin-Tripp & Mitchell-Kernan, 1977).

Egocentrism seems better used as a description of particular pieces of writing, rather than of children in particular stages of development. Children's texts are often egocentric in their lack of connectedness, paucity of details, inadequacy, or incompleteness of references. These texts do not seem to take the perspective of the reader,

nor realize the needs of a reader. It often seems that the child is incapable of directing the flow of information and disregards or is unaware of whether the message is being received.

Text

While the notion of egocentrism may help describe these texts, it is equally useful to return to the source of writing in inner speech and, ultimately, in dialogue. Many early texts are written as if they were the child's part of a dialogue with the reader. The influence of dialogue on children's writing can also be seen in the abundance of dialogue in early writing. Teachers seem to feel dialogue must be taught later in school when punctuation is stressed. However, children come early and naturally to dialogue because it is the source for their writing. Some teachers recognize the importance of dialogue and the aid to early writing in external speech. They will often encourage discussions as a prewriting exercise. (See Rosen & Rosen, 1973, on the use of play and drama.)

Gundlach et al. (1979) have found that while a child may produce an egocentric text, the same child may produce one which shows a shrewd sense of audience. Then the task becomes to determine under what circumstances a child will produce such texts. Further examination shows that children can manipulate all three aspects of the composing process, but not always at the same time. Topic, text, and reader are all present from the beginning; but the young writer cannot deal with them all at once. Many mature writers cannot either; some write in three stages: (a) write about a topic, (b) rewrite

86

with a particular audience in mind, and (c) revise the text. Similarly, it is easier to get children to write in stages as well, not demanding everything at once.

Rosen and Rosen (1973) note:

It doesn't take long with a six or seven-year-old to observe that if he is interrupted in his flow of thought he finds difficulty in reading through what he has written and in picking up the lost thought. (p. 150)

Even older children find it difficult to switch from writer to reader, even if not done in successive stages. Textual editing, which requires simultaneously monitoring for ideas, mechanical errors, as well as information missing for a reader, is an

---

It is artificial to isolate subject, text, and reader, even though clinicians and teachers may temporarily do so to help children write.

---

impossible and incomprehensible task for most beginning writers.

As a word of caution, it is artificial to isolate subject, text, and reader, even though clinicians and teachers may temporarily do so to help children to write. Only certain subjects are appropriate for given modes of discourse, which in turn are only appropriate for certain audiences, and which will produce specific textual structures. For example, within the mode of discourse of correspondence, the text of a letter will change considerably depending on the relationship between writer and reader. Even in the same letter, topic will have an effect (e.g., discussion of a family incident

versus directions for a trip). A piece of writing is a product of a complex process of writing that depends on the activity of composing. One can no more separate its parts than one can lettering from symbolizing (Moffett, 1979) although one may want to understand the different aspects of this process to help beginning writers who are experiencing difficulty with writing.

CONCLUSION

The complexity of writing, beyond its dependence on oral language and reading, creates many problems for specific children which can be called a writing disability (sometimes, a written language problem). For example, underlying processing capacities of attention and memory, as well as levels of cognitive and logical functioning, are required in additional ways for this new activity. Certainly, disabilities that have impeded children in earlier development may reemerge in writing. Coming as it does at the end of a long line of developmental achievements and dependent on these for functioning, it is not surprising to find many disabled children who also display written language problems. Not all disorders at lower levels will surface in writing and also writing may prove beneficial in remediation of other disorders (Johnson & Myklebust, 1967). Once the nature of writing and the demands it makes as an activity on the child are clearly understood, it should be expected that specific writing disorders will be found.

One way to look at a child's performance on a task is to ask: (a) what capacities or abilities or competencies does the child bring to the task, and (b) what demands does the task make on the child? Unless a task is a repetition of one previously performed by the child, there will be some new elements of demand. In performing the task the child demonstrates his or her already acquired capacities as well as the ability to master new demands. The mastery of these tasks becomes part of the child's competencies. This process of the enlarging of an individual's capabilities is familiar to educators from teaching situations, but it is also evident in other performance situations (e.g., in assessment). For example, the subtest on many intelligence quotient (IQ) measures which asks for verbal definitions is considered to assess verbal intelligence. Such definitional tasks measure the ability to use verbal knowledge within the demands of definition-making (Litowitz, 1977). Different demands will be made on verbal knowledge if measured on a freer, nondefinitional, verbal expression task or on a receptive picture-labeling recognition task. However, once definition-making is acquired, this capacity will become part of verbal knowledge to be used in meeting new task demands, such as making texts (Bruner & Olson, 1978; Olson, 1977).

Similarly in writing tasks, when a child is shown a picture (e.g., Picture Story Language Text, Myklebust, 1965), a series of pictures (e.g., Test of Written Language, Hammill & Larsen, 1978) or asked to write an autobiography (e.g., Weiner, 1980), the written performance will be different because the differing tasks make differential demands on the child's underlying capabilities. Other factors such as who asks the child to write, whom does the child envision will be the reader, what are the instructions, who chooses the picture, and what is the topic will also affect the product.

Therefore in every assessment it is necessary to determine underlying capacities, demands of the specific activity, and specific task demands. The division of disabilities in writing into two groups is meant to facilitate such an evaluation by careful discussion of underlying abilities or processes and of the additional demands of writing per se. A better understanding of these should help in determining how they interact in a specific writing task. A particular piece of writing can only be evaluated in light of this kind of information. Multiple frameworks are needed from which to evaluate the activity of writing: what the writer brings to the activity; the nature of the activity; and the product of that activity.

REFERENCES

Anglin, J. *Word, object and conceptual development.* New York: W.W. Norton, 1977.

Applebee, A. *The child's concept of story.* Chicago: University of Chicago Press, 1978.

Beers, J.W., & Henderson, E.H. A study of developing orthographic concepts among first graders. *Research in the Teaching of English,* 1977, *11,* 133–148.

Britton, J. Teaching writing. In A. Davies (Ed.), *Problems of language and learning.* London: Heinemann, 1975.

Britton, J., Burgess, T., Martin, N., McLeod, A., & Rosen, J. *The development of writing abilities (11–18).* Middlesex, England: Macmillan Education Ltd., 1975.

Brown, R. A new paradigm of reference. In G. Miller & E. Lenneberg (Ed.), *Psychology and biology of language and thought.* New York: Academic Press, 1978.

Bruner, J.S. *Beyond the information given.* New York: W.W. Norton & Co., 1973.

Bruner, J.S. Language as an instrument of thought. In A.

88

Davies (Ed.), *Problems of language and learning.* London: Heinemann, 1975.

Bruner, J.S., & Olson, D. Symbols and texts as tools of intellect. *Interchange.* (Ontario Institute for Studies in Education.) 1978, *8*, (4), 1–15.

Chao, Y.R. *Language and symbolic systems.* London: Cambridge University Press, 1970.

de Saussure, F. *Course in general linguistics.* New York: Philosophical Library, 1959. (Original: Cours de linguistique generale. Payot: Paris. 1916).

Dever, R.B. *Teaching the American language to kids.* Columbus, Ohio: Charles E. Merrill, 1978.

Downing, J.A. *The initial teaching alphabet: Reading experiment.* Glenview, Ill.: Scott, Foresman, 1965.

Ervin-Tripp, S., & Mitchell-Kernan, C. *Child discourse.* New York: Academic Press, 1977.

Fillmore, C. *Santa Cruz lectures on Deixis: 1971.* Bloomington, Ind.: Indiana University Linguistics Club, 1975.

Gardner, H. *Artful scribbles.* New York: Basic Books, 1980.

Geest, T. van der, Gerstel, R., Appel, R., & Tervoort, B.Th. *The Child's communicative competence: Language capacity in three groups of children from different social classes.* The Hague: Mouton, 1973.

Gelb, I.J. *A study of writing* (2nd Ed.). Chicago: University of Chicago Press, 1963.

Gibson, E., & Levin, H. *The psychology of reading.* Cambridge, Mass.: M.I.T. Press, 1975.

Gundlach, R.A., Litowitz, B.E., & Moses, R.A. The ontogenesis of the writer's sense of audience: Rhetorical theory and children's written discourse. In R.L. Brown & M. Steinman (Eds.) *Rhetoric 78.* Minneapolis: University of Minnesota Center for Advanced Studies on Language, Style and Literary Theory, 1979.

Halliday, M.A., & Hasan, R. *Cohesion in English.* London: Longman Group Ltd., 1976.

Hammill, D.D., & Larsen, S.C. *Test of written language* (TOWL). Austin, Tex: Pro-Ed, 1978.

Harris, M.M. Oral and written syntax attainment of second graders. *Research in the Teaching of English.* 1977, *11*, 117–132.

Hildreth, G. Developmental sequences in name writing. *Child Development*, 1936, *7*, 291–303.

Hunt, K. Recent measures in syntactic development. In S.C. Larson (Ed.), *Children and writing in the elementary school.* New York: Oxford University Press, 1975.

Jakobson, R. Linguistics and poetics. In T. Sebeok (Ed.), *Style in language.* New York: John Wiley & Sons, 1960.

Johnson, D., & Myklebust, H. *Learning disabilities: Educational principles and practices.* New York: Grune & Stratton, 1967.

Kellogg, R., & O'Dell, S. *The psychology of children's art.* New York: Random House, 1967.

Litowitz, B.E. Learning to make definitions. *Journal of Child Language.* 1977, *4*, 289–304.

Loban, W.D. *The language of elementary school children.* NCTE Research Report #1. Champaign, Ill.: National Center for Teachers of English, 1964.

Lopate, P. The transition from speech to writing. In B. Zavatsky & R. Padgett (Eds.), *The whole word catalogue 2.* New York: McGraw-Hill, 1977.

Luria, A.R. Dynamic approach to the mental development of an abnormal child. In *World Health Organization: Seminar on the mental health of the subnormal child.* Milan: WHO, 1959.

Luria, A.R. The development of writing in the child. In M. Cole (Ed.), *Selected writings of A.R. Luria.* White Plains, N.Y.: M.E. Sharpe, 1978.

Lyons, J. *Introduction to theoretical linguistics.* London: Cambridge University Press, 1968.

Mandler, J.M., & Johnson, N.S. Remembrance of things parsed: Story structure and recall. *Cognitive Psychology*, 1977, *9*, 111–151.

Meyer, B. *The organization of prose and its effects on memory.* Amsterdam: Elsevier North-Holland Publishing Co., 1975.

Moffett, J. *Teaching the universe of discourse.* Boston: Houghton Mifflin, 1968.

Moffett, J. Integrity in the teaching of writing. *Phi Delta Kappan*, December 1979. pp. 276–279.

Myklebust, H. *Development and disorders of written language.* Vol. 1. New York: Grune & Stratton, 1965.

Myklebust, H. *Development and disorders of written language.* Vol. 2. New York: Grune & Stratton, 1973.

O'Donnell, R.C. A critique of some indices of syntactic maturity. *Research in the Teaching of English*, 1976, *10*, 31–38.

O'Donnell, R.C., Griffin, W.J., & Norris, R.C. *The syntax of kindergarten and elementary school children: A transformational analysis.* NCTE Research Report #8. Champaign, Ill.: National Council of Teachers of English, 1967.

Olson, D. From utterance to text: The bias of language in speech and writing. *Harvard Educational Review*, 1977, *47*, 257–281.

Piaget, J. *Judgment and reasoning in the child.* New York: Routledge & Kegan Paul, 1951. (Original: 1924).

Piaget, J. *The language and thought of the child.* New York: Meridian Books, 1955. (Original: 1923).

Piaget, J., & Inhelder, B. *The psychology of the child.* New York: Basic Books, 1969.

Read, C. Pre-school children's knowledge of English phonology. *Harvard Educational Review*, 1971, *41*, 1–34.

Read, C. Lessons to be learned from the preschool orthographer. In E. Lenneberg & E. Lenneberg (Eds.), *Foundations of language development: A multidisci-*

plinary approach. Vol. 2. New York: Academic Press, 1975.

Rosen, C., & Rosen, H. *The language of primary school children.* Middlesex, England: Penguin Books Ltd., 1973.

Rousseau, J.J. *Essai sur l'origine des langes.* Paris: Bibliotheque du Graphe, 1817. A. Belin edition 1817. (Original: 1761).

Shaughnessy, M.P. *Errors and expectations: A guide for the teacher of basic writing.* New York: Oxford University Press, 1977.

Stein, N.L., & Nezworski, M.T. The effect of organization and instructional set on story memory. *Discourse Processes,* 1978, *1,* 177–193.

Thorndyke, P.W. Cognitive structures in comprehension and memory of narrative discourse. *Cognitive Psychology,* 1977, *9,* 77–110.

Villiers, J.G. de, & Villiers, P.A. de. *Language acquisition.* Cambridge, Mass.: Harvard University Press, 1978.

Vygotsky, L.S. *Thought and language.* Cambridge, Mass.: M.I.T. Press, 1962. (Original: 1934).

Vygotsky, L.S. *Mind in society: The development of higher psychological processes.* Cambridge, Mass.: Harvard University Press, 1978.

Weigl, E. On written language: Its acquisition and its alexic-agraphic disturbances. In E. Lenneberg & E. Lenneberg (Eds.), *Foundations of language development: A multidisciplinary approach.* Vol. 2. New York: Academic Press, 1975.

Weiner, E. Diagnostic evaluation of writing skills. *Journal of Learning Disabilities,* 1980, *13,* 48–53.

Zaporozhets, A.V., & Elkonin, D.B. *The psychology of preschool children.* Cambridge, Mass.: M.I.T. Press, 1971.

Improving Written Expression in Learning Disabled Students

Rita Silverman, Ph.D.
Assistant Professor
Department of Education
Rutgers College
New Brunswick, New Jersey

Naomi Zigmond, Ph.D.
Professor
Special Education Program
University of Pittsburgh
Pittsburgh, Pennsylvania

Judith M. Zimmerman, Ed.D.
Assistant Professor
Department of Education
Rutgers College
New Brunswick, New Jersey

Ada Vallecorsa, Ph.D.
Assistant Professor
Special Education Program
University of North Carolina
*   at Greensboro*
Greensboro, North Carolina

ELEMENTARY AND SECONDARY schools have always been concerned that students become literate, but most of the contemporary pressures on schools have stressed the urgency of helping children to read rather than write. The purpose of this article is to begin to redress this imbalance by offering some practical suggestions about ways in which learning disabled (LD) students of all ages can be encouraged to write.

It is fundamental to human growth and development that individuals become competent in various forms of expression. Language is basic to communication, and writing is perhaps the most sophisticated form of language. It depends almost entirely on three other forms—talking, listening, and reading—but it involves distinctive skills that set it apart. Motor skills are required to produce the graphic images, and stored memories of motor patterns for cursive and manuscript letters must be reviewed. Spelling skills are required with easy recall of both regular

0271-8294/81/0012-0091$2.00
© 1981 Aspen Systems Corporation

92

sound-symbol associations and irregular or nonphonetic ones. Syntactical competence is required, including knowledge of the conventions of punctuation, capitalization, usage, and so on.

Writing is often used as a generic term that encompasses the entire expressive, graphic process, including generation of ideas, spelling, syntax, and penmanship. The focus of this article will be on writing as the communication of ideas.

ASSESSMENT OF WRITING ABILITIES

Children with learning disabilities are one group of children who have serious problems with writing. Some educators would suggest that the written language problems of these students are merely reflections of subtle but pervasive oral language problems that include deficits in perceiving, interpreting, formulating, and producing spoken language (Wiig & Semel, 1980). Others (Myklebust, 1973) find that the poor written expression among these students is an inevitable consequence of reading disabilities. Still others would suggest that an inability to write may appear as a specific learning disability in the absence of other language disorders. For example, Vallett (1969) includes the ability to express oneself through written language as one of the 53 separate learning behaviors that may be deficient in students who have learning disabilities.

This latter notion, that an LD student may have a specific disorder of written expression, has gained widespread acceptance since the publication of operational criteria for determining the presence of a learning disability in the *Federal Register* (1977). The announcement that a significant discrepancy between intellectual potential and actual performance on some measure of written expression could be sufficient grounds for labeling a child as learning disabled sparked a new interest in assessment of written language and in the development and publication of new tests of written expressive abilities. The Test of Written Language (TOWL) (Hammill & Larsen, 1978) and the Diagnostic Evaluation of Writing Skills (DEWS) (Weiner, 1980) have appeared in recent years as supplements or replacements for older tests already in use (e.g., Picture Story Language Test, Myklebust, 1965).

TEACHING WRITTEN LANGUAGE

Although the assessment of written expressive abilities is now receiving some attention in learning disabilities literature, the teaching of written language remains a virtually ignored area. A review of "methods" textbooks designed for teachers of learning disabled or mildly handicapped students indicates that this topic is given only minimal coverage. Faas (1980) devotes 60 pages of a 400-page text to diagnosis and remediation of spelling and handwriting problems but is not concerned with problems of written expression of ideas. Johnson and Morasky (1980) discuss remedial approaches to oral language problems, reading problems, arithmetic problems, and perceptual-motor problems with no mention of written composition throughout their text. In similar fashion, Wiig and Semel (1980), Lerner (1971), Wallace and Kauffman (1978), and Hammill and Bartel (1978) seem to ignore the area of remediation of written expression of ideas.

The same trend is reflected in the learning disabilities classroom. In a recent study of 11 self-contained learning disabilities classrooms, Leinhardt, Zigmond, and Cooley (1980) observed how 105 LD students spent their time. Among the student and teacher behaviors that were recorded, there were two categories of writing behavior: (a) copying, or transcribing written material generated by the teacher or printed in a book or workbook, and (b) creating written output, or writing words, sentences, or paragraphs generated by the student. Using data collected during 30 hours of observation spread over 20 weeks of schooling, they found that students spent an average of about 25 minutes of each 270-minute day in writing activities, but that 75% of this time, or 19 minutes per day, was spent *copying*. This included such activities as copying the morning news from the blackboard, copying letters or words in a handwriting exercise, writing spelling words 10 times each, copying sentences from book to worksheet, or rewriting corrected work. They found that students who were beginning readers spent less than 5 minutes per day in generating written language, which consisted mostly of thinking up single words to fill in the blanks on a ditto or worksheet. Even students who could read at the second-, third-, or fourth-grade levels spent an average of only 7.5 minutes per day in creative writing tasks.

Learning disabled students are not the only ones receiving little opportunity to write creatively. A British project (Schools Council, 1975) which examined normal children's writings in all subject areas found that only 5% of all the writing examined encouraged children to express themselves in their own words. Graves (1978) speculated that American children in regular classes spend so little time learning to write and write so little that by the time they graduate from high school they will have lost an important means of thinking. His recent survey of 36 school systems disclosed that second- through sixth-grade students, on the average, wrote only three pieces over a 3-month period (Graves, 1978).

WHAT TO DO?

Although writing is frequently talked about (Why Johnny Can't Write, *Newsweek*, December 8, 1977) and cited as a priority area for instructional emphasis in both regular and special education (Larsen & Poplin, 1980; Mellon, 1976), it seldom seems to be practiced in the schools.

Some of the responsibility for the limited amount of time currently devoted to writing may be traced to the attitudes of the teachers who first introduce the subject of writing to children and to the educational system which produced the teachers. These teachers seldom look forward to the idea of teaching writing. Most of them do not write themselves; they do not like to write; they feel they are poor writers. Most report that they lack time to write because of work

94

demands or that they do not believe it is necessary to practice writing to teach writing (Graves, 1978). Furthermore, most teachers are inadequately trained to teach writing. Graves' random survey of 30 universities revealed 169 courses in reading, 30 courses in literature, and only 2 courses in writing (Graves, 1978). Teachers generally lack the background or experience to teach writing.

Nevertheless there can be little doubt about the converging research evidence that children learn what they spend time doing (Barr, 1980; Blake, 1971; Brown & Saks, 1980; Evertson, 1980; Fillmer, 1968; Fisher, Filby, Marliave, Cahen, Dishaw, Moore, & Berliner, 1978; Fox, 1976; Leinhardt et al., 1980; Leonard, 1976; Stallings, 1980; Stallings, Needels, & Stayrook, 1979). Educators cannot be sure how much classroom time *should* be devoted

---

Learning to write requires writing, and writing practice should be a major new emphasis in classrooms for both normal and learning disabled children.

---

to creative writing but undoubtedly learning to write is important, learning to write requires writing, and writing practice should be a major new emphasis in classrooms for both normal and LD children.

Teachers must overcome their anxiety about teaching writing and find new ways to engage students in creative writing tasks, paying particular attention to how the writing assignment is presented and how it is responded to by the teacher (Burhans, 1968; Daly & Miller, 1975; Gee,

1970; Groff, 1975; Rohman & Wiecke, 1964; Stevens, 1973).

Presenting creative writing tasks: The prewriting phase

How teachers introduce the written language assignment affects the students' writing performance. Several researchers have noted that oral language development is a prerequisite to effective written communication.

Language is basic to communication (Allen, 1976). It enables children to develop abstract thought (Bruner, Goodnow, & Austin, 1956; Piaget, 1974). Loban (1963) reported that if children's oral language and cognitive development were restricted, they would be unable to produce disciplined, well-organized, and logical compositions. Loban and others (Emig, 1971; Graves, 1978; Parker, 1972) emphasize the value of involving students in oral language experiences prior to the writing tasks. This prewriting phase includes time to talk about what is to be written and to discuss the ideas with other people. Miller and Ney (1968) reported that students who participated in systematic oral language exercises wrote with greater freedom and facility. Waldschmidt (1973) found that student writing performance and attitude improved significantly with a talk-write approach. Maxwell and Hook (reported in Porter, 1972) agreed that student-to-student oral exchange encouraged personal and imaginative writing.

The evidence seems clear. If the teacher structures the presentation of the written assignment with prewriting activities which involve time to think, to experience, to discuss, and to interact with language, this is likely to have a positive effect on written language achievement.

Presenting creative writing tasks: The writing phase

Expressive language usually involves the free flow of ideas and feelings in natural, unstructured ways. Expressive writing tasks often take the form of journals, diaries, spontaneous responses, informal essays, unstructured monologues, impressions, and personal letters. But to students not used to expressing themselves, an unstructured request for written output like "What did you do over summer vacation?", even when preceded by oral discussion of the topic, can often yield little more than severe anxiety and blank tablets. "Writer's block" in students can be overcome by offering students who are new to generative writing some organizers or cues to be used during the writing task itself. During the prewriting phase, in the oral discussion of the writing topic, teacher and students together generate questions which will be answered by the written output. During the writing phase, students organize their creative writing to answer these questions. This technique has been used successfully, even with middle school LD students who were not only poor readers but who also had histories of being unable to write. The following are a series of questions generated around the creative writing assignment: Writing a commercial or advertisement for a make-believe product.

1. What is the name of your product?
2. What is it made of?
3. Why is it good? What does it do?
4. Why is it better than similar products?
5. How much does it cost? Where can I buy one?

Two compositions produced using these organizers follow.

Presenting the All-Pro Football by J.H. Football Co.

The All-Pro Football is made from leather. It is shaped like a lemon, has leather strings and comes in all colors.

Our dynamite football weighs less than the regular more expensive footballs. It travels further when thrown and it lasts longer because the leather is very thick.

Our product is guaranteed to stick to your hands because of our secret treatment on the leather. When our ball is kicked or thrown it will travel like a bullet, never going off target. It will not blow up if punctured by steel, glass, or under heavy pressure, and this dynamite ball can be used on any surface.

You can buy our football for the low price of $25.00. Our football can be purchased in all sporting goods stores around the world.

Introducing the new Pinto cars by A.P. Pinto Co.

Our car's body is constructed of chrome and the frame is made of heavy duty steel. The Pinto can get you from place to place, while giving you 37 m.p.g. that sets the pace. It has comfortable leather seats for five, AM/FM radio, air conditioning, slit racing mags, and a four-speed stick shift.

Our car has a lifetime guarantee on all parts and labor. When you come in our showroom you may test drive for 2 or 3 weeks; if you don't like it, you may return it. Also, when you test drive our car you will receive an A.P. Pinto bumper sticker. Come on in and see our new sports car. And you can take it home for the low, low, low, low price of $3,420.06.

96

These students had never written a composition before. They had always avoided written assignments and because they were only second-grade readers in sixth grade, their teachers had given up demanding written responses. But both boys responded well to the prewriting discussion and to the questions printed on a ditto which they kept with them while they wrote. The questions served not only as organizers for the responses, but also as reminders of the answers they had given during the oral discussion. The question made the task much easier to complete.

A second set of questions generated for an assignment required students to describe how it felt to be some inanimate object.

1. What do you look like?
2. What do you see (as you start out; where you are; who or what is around you; etc.)?
3. Who comes to get you? What do they do to get you ready?
4. How do you feel when you're moving fast or slow?
5. Tell about something that happened to you while moving (exciting, sad, funny, etc.).
6. How do you feel when they put you away or when they've finished with you?

The following compositions are further examples of products written by middle school LD students using this technique. The imaginative and humorous quality of the compositions is obvious. These students would not have been able to write these ideas had it not been for the organizers provided them throughout the process.

How would it feel?

I am round and I have Chocolate Chips in me and I come from the chocolate chip mine. There they are always putting chips in us all the time. I can see a lot of other chocolate chip cookies, and here comes the baker with a big blue bag. The baker wants us to meet a friend of his, Cookie Man! Once we got to the store, I saw a little boy and he came over to read about our friend cookie man and when he grabbed the bag he broke our other friend, Juan.

Suddenly he shook the bag and I hit the side and lost all my chips. He threw us in the cart and I hit a can and then he threw a loaf of bread on us. We were lucky because it was soft. When we got to the boy's house he took me out of the bag and got some milk and dunked me in it and then he took a big bite out of me with a Crunch!

What it would feel like to be a piece of chalk

Hi, I'm a piece of chalk. I am long and skinny and my color is white. Usually I just sit here in the chalk rack waiting for someone to pick me up. Other pieces of chalk are around me in the tray, too. Some of them are yellow and some of them are red. They're all skinny just like me but some of them are real short and look all worn out. They're not all new like I am. I can see kids coming into the Learning Lab from my seat up here. Some of them are making lots of noise and clowning while they are picking up their work folders. Usually the teacher tells them to be quiet and get started working. The teacher is the one who uses me most. But sometimes the kids write things on the board with me too. Sometimes they use me to write spelling words or solve math problems. Once they even used me to write "Goodbye, Mr. Hubbard, we will miss you" when our student teacher left us. I like it best when they write long words with me because then I know I am really working hard. But I don't like it when people move me along too slow. When they do that I make screeching noises to let them know they should go faster. This usually makes everyone cover up their ears. Once someone dropped me on the floor and I almost broke into a lot of pieces. That's what happened to my friend, Juan. He broke into 4 little pieces that were too small for anyone to use. Now he just sits here collecting dust. When they finish using me and put me away I usually check to see how much of me is left. The smaller I get the better I feel, because it means I have been useful.

In all writing assignments, students were told not to be concerned about punctuation, grammatical correctness, or spelling; those elements of the writing process would be dealt with at a later time. Students were to concentrate *only* on ideas and were to be as creative and imaginative as possible. Therefore the samples presented here were edited by teachers and students in all areas but creativity.

Once students experienced success with written expression, the teacher's role in developing organizers and cues could be faded slowly; students learned to develop organizers themselves if they needed them. In a matter of months students began to attack a blank piece of paper and a writing assignment with courage, if not with ease.

Presenting creative writing tasks: The postwriting phase

As with most forms of expression, writing will not flourish unless it gives the child some form of satisfaction. Initially, the fact that the writing exists, that it is finished, may be enough to make the writer feel the effort to produce it has been worthwhile. But such satisfactions are short-lived unless the work evokes some response on the part of others. Few want to go on writing unless the end product attracts attention. (Sealey, Sealey, & Millmore, 1979, p. 2)

Most research indicates that students respond favorably and with more enthusiasm for continued writing when rewarded with praise instead of criticism. Yet most teachers still return creative writing assignments to students filled with red-penned corrections of spelling, mechanics, and punctuation. Research evidence confirms that this is probably a bad practice. Groff (1975) has found that although positive or negative criticism did not affect the quality of students' writing, it did affect student attitudes toward writing. Both Stevens (1973) and Gee (1970) concluded that comments of praise were more effective than negative comments or no comments at all when promoting positive attitudes toward writing.

Teachers must learn to respond to creative writing attempts with positive comments on the content of the assignment and suggestions for improvement of thought organization and presentation. Rough drafts should be encouraged in which attention is paid only to ideas, with errors in mechanics, penmanship, and spelling ignored. Only after the student has received positive reinforcement for free expression of ideas should the teacher and student critique the other aspects of the composition, to ready it for final form.

98   CONCLUSIONS

The mandate to improve written language skills is not new. Five years ago, the National Council of Teachers of English (1975) called public attention to the fact that students' writing ability seemed to be diminishing over time. The renewed emphasis on "the basics" has led to an increase in time spent developing vocabulary, spelling, reading, and math, yet students still seem to be writing less and less. Because written expression of ideas is an important skill, the trend must be reversed.

Research has demonstrated repeatedly that what children learn from their classroom experiences is a function of what they do during class. This article has provided some data to confirm that children in school today spend far too little time practicing expression of their ideas in written form.

Teachers in both basic education and special education should allocate more time to creative writing. Some directions for planning and implementing creative writing tasks have been provided. Writing is a little like playing the piano: "talent always is involved, but so is practice, for only through practice is talent honed, refined and finished" (Leonard, 1976, p. 59).

REFERENCES

Allen, R.V. *Language experiences in communication.* Boston: Houghton Mifflin, 1976.

Barr, R. *School, class, group and pace effects on learning.* Paper presented at the annual meeting of the American Education Research Association, Boston, April 1980.

Blake, H.E. Written composition in English primary schools. *Elementary English,* 1971, 48, 605–615.

Brown, B.W., & Saks, D.H. *The allocation and use of instructional time in reading and mathematics: Some theory and evidence.* Paper presented at the annual meeting of the American Education Research Association, Boston, April 1980.

Bruner, J., Goodnow, J., & Austin, G. *A study of thinking.* New York: John Wiley & Sons, 1956.

Burhans, C.S. *Extended testing of a unified experimental course in composition in a variety of materials and formats.* U.S. Office of Education Cooperative Research Project No. 7-1149. Lansing, Mich.: Michigan State University, 1968.

Criteria for determining the existence of a specific learning disability. *Federal Register,* 42 (250), Thursday, December 29, 1977, 65083, Section 121 a. 541.

Daly, J.A., & Miller, M.D. Apprehension of writing as a predictor of message intensity. *The Journal of Psychology,* 1975, 89, 175–177.

Emig, J. *The composing process of 12th graders.* National Council of Teachers of English, Research Report No. 13. Champaign, Ill.: NCTE, 1971.

Evertson, C. *Differences in instructional activities in high and low achieving junior high classes.* Paper presented at the annual meeting of the American Education Research Association, Boston, April 1980.

Faas, L.A. *Children with learning problems.* Boston: Houghton Mifflin, 1980.

Fillmer, H.T. Teaching composition through literature. *Elementary English,* 1968, 45, 736–739.

Fisher, C.W., Filby, N.N., Marliave, R., Cahen, L.S., Dishaw, M.M., Moore, J.E., & Berliner, D.C. *Teacher behaviors, academic learning time and student achievement: Final report of Phase III-B, Beginning teacher evaluation study.* Technical Report V-1. San Francisco, Calif.: Far West Laboratory for Educational Research and Development, 1978.

Fox, P. Why Johnny can't and the cat in the hat. *English Journal,* 1976, 65, 38–39.

Gee, T.C. *The effects of written comment on expository composition.* Doctoral dissertation, North Texas State University, 1970. (University Microfilms No. 71-551)

Graves, D. *Balance the basics: Let them write.* New York: Ford Foundation, 1978.

Groff, P. Does negative criticism discourage children's composition? *Language Arts,* 1975, 52, 1032–1033.

Hammill, D.D., & Bartel, N.R. *Teaching children with learning or behavior problems* (2nd ed.). Boston: Allyn & Bacon, 1978.

Hammill, D., & Larsen, S. *Test of written language*. Austin, Tex.: Pro-Ed., 1978.

Johnson, S.W., & Morasky, R.L. *Learning disabilities* (2nd ed.). Boston: Allyn & Bacon, 1980.

Larsen, S.C., & Poplin, M.S. *Methods for educating the handicapped*. Boston: Allyn & Bacon, 1980.

Leinhardt, G., Zigmond, N., & Cooley, W.W. *Reading instruction and its effects*. Paper presented at the annual meeting of the American Educational Research Associates, Boston, April 1980.

Leonard, M.H. Practice makes better: Notes on a writing program. *English Journal*, September 1976, *65*, 59–63.

Lerner, J.W. *Children with learning disabilities*. Boston: Houghton Mifflin, 1971.

Loban, W. *The language of elementary school children*. National Council of Teachers of English Research Report No. 1. Champaign, Ill.: NCTE, 1963.

Mellon, J.C. Round two of the national writing assessment—Interpreting the apparent decline of writing ability: A review. *Research in the Teaching of English*, September 1976, *10*, 67–74.

Miller, B.D., & Ney, J.W. The effects of systematic oral exercises on the writing of fourth-grade students. *Research in the Teaching of English*, 1968, *2*, 44–61.

Myklebust, H. *Development and disorders of written language: Picture story language test* (Vol. 1). New York: Grune & Stratton, 1965.

Myklebust, H. *Development and disorders of written language: Studies of normal and exceptional children* (Vol. 2). New York: Grune & Stratton, 1973.

National Council of Teachers of English. Composition: A position statement. *Elementary English*, February 1975, *52*, 194–196.

Parker, R.P. Jr. Focus in the teaching of writing: On process or product. *English Journal*, 1972, *61*(9), 1328–1333.

Piaget, J. *The language and thought of the child*. New York: New American Library, 1974.

Porter, J. Research report. *Elementary English*, 1972, *49*(6), 863–870.

Rohman, D.G., & Wiecke, A.O. *Pre-writing: The construction and application of models for concept formation in writing*. U.S. Office of Education Cooperative Research Project No. 2174. East Lansing, Mich.: Michigan State University, 1964.

Schools Council. *Why writing*. London: Institute of Education, 1975.

Sealey, L., Sealey, N., & Millmore, M. *Children's writing: An approach for the primary grades*. Newark, Del.: International Reading Association, 1979.

Stallings, J.A. *Allocated academic learning time revisited, or beyond time on task*. Paper presented at the annual meeting of the American Educational Research Association, Boston, April 1980.

Stallings, J.A., Needels, M., & Stayrook, N. *The teaching of basic reading skills in secondary schools, Phase I and Phase III*. Menlo Park, Calif.: SRI International, 1979.

Stevens, A.E. *The effects of positive and negative evaluation on the written composition of low performing high school students*. Doctoral dissertation, Boston University, 1973. (University Microfilms No. 73-23, 617)

Vallet, R.E. *Programming learning disabilities*. Belmont, Calif.: Fearon-Pitman Publishers, 1969.

Waldschmidt, E. *Pilot studies in composition: Their effects upon students and participating English teachers*. Unpublished doctoral dissertation, University of Illinois, 1973.

Wallace, G., & Kauffman, J.M. *Teaching children with learning problems*. Columbus, Ohio: Charles E. Merrill, 1978.

Weiner, E.S. The diagnostic evaluation of writing skills (DEWS): Application of DEWS criteria to writing samples. *Learning Disabilities Quarterly*, 1980, *3*(2), 54–55.

Why Johnny can't write. *Newsweek*, December 8, 1977.

Wiig, E.H., & Semel, E.M. *Language assessment and intervention for the learning disabled*. Columbus, Ohio: Charles E. Merrill, 1980.

Notices

NEW YORK STATE SPEECH-LANGUAGE-HEARING ASSOCIATION CONVENTION

The annual convention of the New York State Speech-Language-Hearing Association will be held April 12 through April 15 at the Nevele Country Club in Ellenville, New York. For information contact: Ellen Morris Tiegerman, 86-39 105 Street, Richmond Hills, NY 11418.

Notices featured in TLD include information on upcoming events and other areas of interest. Please address all material to be considered for publication in Notices to: Editor, Notices, TLD, Aspen Systems Corporation, 1600 Research Boulevard, Rockville MD 20850.